Ending Nurse-to-Nurse Hostility

WHY NURSES EAT THEIR YOUNG AND EACH OTHER

Kathleen Bartholomew, RN, MN

with Foreword by Sandra P. Thomas, PhD, RN, FAAN

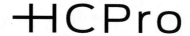

Kathleen Bartholomew, RN, MN, Author
Amanda Waddell, Editor
Jean St. Pierre, Director of Operations
Lauren Rubenzahl, Copy Editor
Jackie Diehl Singer, Graphic Artist

Shane Katz, Cover Designer
Patrick Campagnone, Cover Designer
Daniel Hallett, Cover Photographer
Emily Sheahan, Group Publisher

Advice given is general. Readers should consult professional counsel for specific legal, ethical, or clinical questions.

Arrangements can be made for quantity discounts.

For more information, contact

HCPro, Inc.
P.O. Box 1168
Marblehead, MA 01945
Telephone: 800/650-6787 or 781/639-1872
Fax: 781/639-2982
E-mail: *customerservice@hcpro.com*

Visit HCPro at its World Wide Web sites:
www.hcpro.com and www.hcmarketplace.com

CONTENTS

Dedication vii

Acknowledgements vii

About the author. viii

Foreword ix

Learning objectives. xi

Prologue xiii

Section I: Understanding the forces 1

Chapter one: What is horizontal hostility? 3
    Defining horizontal hostility 3
    Is horizontal hostility intentional? 6
    Tales from the front line 7
    Prevalence 9
    Impact 12
    Retention during a nursing shortage 16
    Summary 18
    Bibliography 19

Chapter two: Exploring theory 23
    Marie's story: A manager's point of view 23
    Oppression theory 25
    Supporting theory: Insights from the animal kingdom. 33
    Populations at risk 34

Figure 2.1: The 10 most frequent forms of lateral violence in
nursing practice 36
Why is horizontal hostility so virulent? 37
Summary 41
Bibliography 42

Chapter three: A root cause analysis of horizontal hostility 45
Marie's search for answers 45
Intrinsic factors 48
Extrinsic factors 58
Summary 66
Bibliography 66

Chapter four: Enlarging the landscape 69
Context is critical 69
Organizational context 70
Professional context 76
In the context of our world 79
Summary 82
Recommended reading 84
Bibliography 84

Section II: Best practices to eliminate horizontal hostility 87
Introduction 89
The big picture: An analogy 92

Chapter five: Nurturing our young 95
Impediments to a healthy new nurse experience 96
Creating a healthy environment for student nurses 98
Figure 5.1: Nurse-to-nurse hostility fact sheet .102
Bringing horizontal hostility to light at nursing schools 105

New resident nurses 108

    Figure 5.2: Expected behaviors of those who call themselves professionals 111

    Figure 5.3: Cueing cards attached to identification badge 112

Summary 114

Recommended reading 115

Bibliography 116

Chapter six: Managerial response **119**

Awareness: Ability to see the problem 120

    Figure 6.1: Sample questionnaire 125

    Figure 6.2: Verbal abuse survey 126

Communication 127

    Figure 6.3: Charge nurse assessment tool 133

Response 144

Persistence and consistency is mandatory 147

Empowering staff 148

Summary 148

Recommended reading 149

Bibliography 149

Chapter seven: Organizational opportunities **151**

Framework for leading organizational change to eliminate hostility 152

Increase a healthy culture 153

Decrease hostility 166

    Figure 7.1: Commitment to coworkers 169

How the system sets up the manager to fail 172

Summary 173

Recommended reading 175

Bibliography 175

Contents

Chapter eight: Individual response **177**

    Starting with ourselves 177

    Transitioning from a closed system to an open system 180

    Bibliography 182

Epilogue **183**

Nursing education instructional guide **185**

    Instructions for obtaining your nursing contact hours .187

    Nursing education exam 188

    Nursing education evaluation 194

Dedication

With great admiration and love to all of the 9 East Orthopedics and 10 East Spine staff of Swedish Medical Center in Seattle.

Acknowledgements

This book would not have been possible without the years of dedicated research by Sandra Thomas, RN, PhD, FAAN, and Gerald Farrell, RN, PhD. Their work stands out among that of many others as providing the much-needed research that is the foundation of this book.

With great appreciation, I acknowledge Genevieve Bartol, RN, EdD, AHN-C(P), Elaine Goehner, PhD, RN, CPHQ, Linda Westbrook, RN, PhD, John Nance, JD, Wendy Buenzli, RN, MN, and Kathleen Tate, RN, for their tremendous support, encouragement, and guidance.

About the author

Kathleen Bartholomew, RN, MN, a registered nurse and counselor, uses the power of story from her experience as the manager of a large surgical unit to shed light on the challenges and issues facing nurses today. Her strength is her ability to link the academic world with the practical reality of the hospital. Her objective is to serve as a much-needed voice for nursing today.

Bartholomew has been a national speaker for the nursing profession for the past six years. Recognizing that the culture of an institution is critical to patient safety, she speaks on building community in the workplace and improving nurse-physician relationships. *Speak Your Truth: Proven Strategies for Effective Nurse-Physician Communication* was published in 2005 as her Master's thesis. Both her lectures and her books reflect her passion for and love of nursing.

Foreword

Combining her own extensive real-world experience with careful examination of the theoretical and empirical literature on horizontal hostility, Kathleen Bartholomew delivers a book that is sure to make a positive impact. I heartily welcome the contribution of this book, given my own years of research on this pervasive—and worsening—problem.

Clear in her conviction that this destructive phenomenon must be halted, Bartholomew gives readers the tools to halt it. She explains the etiology of horizontal hostility—which is characteristic of all oppressed groups—and then devotes the bulk of her book to best practices to eliminate the problem. Throughout the book, Bartholomew shares vignettes from her own work life, convincing the reader that she knows what it is like "down in the trenches"—a military metaphor so often used by hospital nurses. Therefore, readers will find her advice credible and practical, as well as compassionate and wise.

This book displays special concern for new nurses, whom we cannot afford to lose from the profession. Given that 60% of newly registered nurses are leaving their first positions within six months because of horizontal hostility[1], we urgently need to develop new ways of nurturing our young (addressed in Chapter 5). Bartholomew also focuses on the nurse manager, who is so often caught in a no-win situation between the demands of upper management and the complaints of subordinates (addressed in Chapter 6). In the final chapters of the book, the responsibility of creating healthy workplace cultures is squarely assigned to senior leaders, as well as to the rank and file.

Bartholomew clearly has great respect for nurses at all levels, and she exhorts us all to begin displaying that kind respect and admiration for one another. Ultimately, that is the solution to the problem of horizontal hostility. I fervently hope to see it solved in my lifetime!

Sandra P. Thomas, PhD, RN, FAAN
Professor and Director, PhD Program in Nursing
University of Tennessee, Knoxville
Knoxville, TN

Endnote

1. Griffin, M, 2004. Teaching cognitive rehearsal as a shield for lateral violence: An intervention for newly licensed nurses. *The Journal of Continuing Education in Nursing* 35(6).

Learning objectives

Define horizontal hostility.

List two overt examples of horizontal hostility from the work setting.

List two covert examples of horizontal hostility from the work setting.

Discuss the impact that horizontal hostility has on 1) the individual and 2) the organization.

Explain the ways in which the current system is designed to support the invisibility of nurses.

List two populations at risk for experiencing horizontal hostility.

State four of the most frequent forms of lateral violence.

Explain why horizontal hostility is so virulent.

Identify two intrinsic forces that play a role in horizontal hostility.

Identify two extrinsic forces that play a role in horizontal hostility.

Explain how the organizational structure enables oppression.

Select two factors that contribute to nurses' stress from the context of our world.

List two impediments to a healthy student or resident nurse experience.

Describe six steps that can be taken to create a healthy environment for student nurses.

Name two signs of which managers should be aware that may indicate that horizontal hostility is taking place.

Explain what is meant by a "twofold approach" to eliminating horizontal hostility.

Select one way in which nurse managers can empower staff.

Identify two strategies to nurture a healthy culture within the organization.

Identify two strategies to decrease hostility within the organization.

Identify two practices or behaviors characteristic of a closed system.

Prologue

Skye is a nursing assistant on our unit. Despite having a bachelor's degree in public health and a 3.9 GPA, she is still number 54 on a waiting list for nursing school. Her goal is to gain experience by working as a nursing assistant and eventually become a nursing instructor. However, the experience she is gaining at our hospital isn't just limited to clinical practice.

On this particular morning, she and I are watching the drama unfold as the charge nurses argue over staffing for the floor. There is no point intervening. It is just a few minutes before 7 a.m., and I have counseled both nurses in the past. Emotions are high, and the nurses are arriving at good decisions for the floor despite their arguments.

Finally, everyone goes into report and Skye looks at me with a puzzled expression. "Why the drama?" she asks. I remember that yesterday Skye worked with two staff nurses who spent the entire shift venting about one another—to everyone on the floor but each other. "Is this what they mean by nurses eating their young and each other?" she asks hesitantly.

I take a deep breath. Horizontal hostility is a complex problem with many facets, and I don't want to gloss it over or turn her off to nursing. I want Skye to truly see and understand the forces that create and maintain this problem. It would be just as much of a disservice to Skye as it would be to nursing not to answer this question thoroughly and honestly. Drawing upon my own experience as a nurse manager, as well as research that has been conducted in the United States and other countries, I turn my answer into a book.

Understanding the forces

What is horizontal hostility?

"Define your terms, and I will speak with you."

—*Voltaire*

Defining horizontal hostility

A literature search on aggression in the workplace produces a potpourri of titles: interactive workplace trauma, anger, horizontal hostility, bullying, verbal abuse, and horizontal or lateral violence. These terms are then discussed within a variety of relationships: nurse-to-doctor, patient-to-nurse, and nurse-to-nurse. Although the literature provides a better understanding of the presence and effect of negative emotions in healthcare settings, the lack of a universal term makes it quite a challenge to integrate the research into one cohesive picture. The following are just some of the definitions used in literature on the subject:

Horizontal violence: "Sabotage directed at coworkers who are on the same level within an organization's hierarchy" (Dunn 2003).

Verbal abuse: "Communication perceived by a person to be a harsh, condemnatory attack, either professional or personal. Language intended to cause distress to a target" (Buback 2004).

The majority of research on aggression in nursing has come from Australia and Great Britain. In these countries, the term "bullying" is used to describe workplace aggression. The definition of bullying shares three elements that come from racial and sexual harassment law. "First, bullying is defined in terms of its effect on the recipient—not the intention of the bully. Secondly, there must be a negative effect on the victim. Thirdly, the bullying behavior must be persistent" (Quine 1999). Bullying is a broad term and includes aggression from superiors, subordinates, and peers in the workplace.

Bullying: "The persistent, demeaning and downgrading of humans through vicious words and cruel acts that gradually undermine confidence and self-esteem" (Adams 1997).

The terms "horizontal violence" and "horizontal hostility" are used to portray aggressive behavior between individuals *on the same power level*, such as nurse-to-nurse and manager-to-manager. Research on anger, aggression, bullying, and verbal abuse is relevant because these behaviors are all ways in which hostility expresses itself. In this book, I will use the term "horizontal hostility," using key points as defined by Gerald Farrell, RN, PhD (see below) and congruent with the elements of harassment law listed above.

Horizontal hostility: A consistent pattern of behavior designed to control, diminish, or devalue a peer (or group) that creates a risk to health and/or safety (Farrell 2005).

Overt and covert behaviors

Horizontal hostility can be physical or verbal. In nursing, verbal aggression is more prevalent. It can include any form of mistreatment, spoken or unspoken, that leaves a person feeling personally or professionally attacked, devalued, or humiliated (Farrell 2005). It can be either overt or covert. Since studies show that the majority of our communication is nonverbal and stress is heightened in ambiguous situations, covert behaviors have the biggest impact.

Overt: Name-calling, bickering, fault-finding, backstabbing, criticism, intimidation, gossip, shouting, blaming, using put-downs, raising eyebrows, etc.

Covert: Unfair assignments, sarcasm, eye-rolling, ignoring, making faces behind someone's back, refusing to help, sighing, whining, refusing to work with someone, sabotage, isolation, exclusion, fabrication, etc.

The following is an example of overt hostility experienced by a fellow nurse:

"I am used to being in a charge nurse position and am now working with recovering patients from the cath lab. The hostility here is thinly veiled. I come into work and say something like, 'Nice day today,' and the charge replies, 'What's that supposed to mean?'

We have really sick patients just fresh out of the cath lab. When the charge nurse told me she was going to take a break, I asked her a few questions so I would have the information I needed to cover. I asked, 'Does 212 have a sheath in?' and the charge nurse said, 'What do you want to know for?' I try to ignore her and just do my job.

When she came back from break I told her all that had happened in her absence—for example, that I taped down the IV in 214. Coldly, she responded, 'That could've waited until I returned.' It's a constant, negative, put-you-down undercurrent that never ends."

Is horizontal hostility intentional?

For more than an hour, Bethany has been recounting examples of horizontal hostility over a 14-year career, which brought her to three different states and through major depression. At the end of the interview, I ask her, "Do you think the nurses knew what they were doing? Were their actions intentional?"

She bristles and responds almost indignantly, "Their actions were very intentional. They knew exactly what they were doing!"

I press further, "But were their actions conscious? Do you think those nurses were aware of the pain they were causing you?"

Bethany pauses and her face softens. "No, they were clueless to the effect of their actions. They never looked past [their actions] to see how another person would feel. What got me was how a person could hate someone they didn't even know."

The above scenario has occurred with dozens of nurses whom I have counseled. The intent of backstabbing, intimidation, fault-finding, etc., is to alienate, attack, or punish a coworker. In every case I have handled, the perpetrators did not realize the effects of their actions. Many believed that they were superior because they were upholding a standard of quality patient care. Only through education, which began by confronting the behavior, did nurses begin to comprehend the full extent of their actions. And when a nurse did "get it," the behavior stopped immediately.

It is difficult to even admit that we could be hurting each other in a profession that has its fundamental roots in caring. Uncovering and discussing horizontal hostility is about as easy as a family acknowledging how damaging it is to live with alcoholism. It is embarrassing and is so remotely removed from our idea of the perfect nurse that we shudder to think that it may be true. In addition, there is an unspoken fear, warranted or not, that acknowledging the problem will make it worse. However, if nursing is to survive, we need an immediate intervention. This intervention starts with listening to the voices in the room— the researchers who have uncovered this behavior, and the nurses who are experiencing the hostility.

Tales from the front line

"Our communication is fraught with indirect aggression, bickering, and fault-finding. It is disheartening to experience the underhanded and devastating ways that nurses attack each other. These rifts divide us and lead us to injure one another."

—*Laura Gasparis Vonfrolio, RN, PhD*

There is nothing as powerful as a story. Stories put the truth out into the world— once a story is shared, you cannot call it back. Stories are a means of truth-telling. If we have had a similar experience, a story resonates with us at the deepest level, and there is comfort and validation as we realize that others share our experience.

At the "Horizontal Violence in the Workplace" conference held by the Oregon chapter of the American Psychiatric Nurses Association in October 2005, I asked participants whether they would be willing to share their stories about hostility in the workplace. I collected a list of names and phone numbers of interested nurses and arranged convenient times to speak to each one by phone. As I listened to the first story, I was shocked at the intensity of aggression the nurse had experienced and by the fact that the continuous verbal abuse had resulted in a suicide attempt. From hospitals and academia to outpatient clinic settings, nurses shared with me their poignant experiences with horizontal hostility. I have incorporated many of these stories, and others I have heard throughout my career, into this book (these quotes appear in italics):

"This is what the group of nurses would do to me: I never sat down for 12 hours. It was horrendous. All I know is that if a group works together for long enough, they keep the others outside."

"The smallest thing would trigger retaliation. [The charge nurse's] refusal to speak was the worst. Once she went 27 days without speaking."

"It was the looks [the preceptor] gave me, like I was stupid. In my whole three months of orientation, I can't think of a single time anyone ever complimented me."

"The orientation nurse was ultimately fired. She started drinking and felt attacked all the time. Everything was her fault, all the time."

As nurses shared their experiences with me, two common themes emerged. First, every single participant was gravely concerned about maintaining anonymity for fear of being identified. Even if the violence had happened ten years ago and had been resolved by the abuser leaving the workplace, *all nurses feared retaliation*. The workplace was still viewed as dangerous, and nurses continued to feel vulnerable. Secondly, no matter what the situation, the stories clearly brought up a lot of emotional pain that was difficult to acknowledge. Like those suffering from post-traumatic stress disorder (PTSD), participants appeared to be reliving their hurt all over again. The air was still thick with feelings of loss and betrayal after the conversations were finished. As stories were coaxed from each nurse, the courage required to tell their stories became obvious. Even to be a witness to another's story was upsetting:

"Survivors have to look the other way . . . or go along with the crowd to survive. You have to take the party line even if you don't believe it."

Research shows that these stories are not isolated events and that the effects of these negative emotions have a serious impact. "Horizontal hostility drains nurses of vitality and undermines institutional attempts to create a satisfied nursing workforce" (Thomas 2003).

Prevalence

On an international level, one in three nurses plans to leave his or her position because of horizontal hostility (McMillan 1995). In 1996, a survey was conducted of more than 1,100 employees of a National Health Service Community Trust in England, which included 396 nurses. The bullied staff reported lower job satisfaction, higher job stress, greater depression and anxiety, and greater intent to leave their job. The bully was a superior in 54% of cases, a peer in 34%, and a subordinate 12% of the time. Thirty percent of respondents in the study stated that they were subjected to aggression "on a daily or near daily basis" (Farrell 1999). A study in the United Kingdom of 4,500 nurses showed that one in six nurses reported that they had experienced workplace mistreatment in the past year and that 33% were intending to leave the workplace because of verbal abuse. Mistreatment by peers accounted for 41% of verbal abuse (Gilmour and Hamlin 2003).

Studies in the United States indicate that 90%–97% of nurses experience verbal abuse from physicians (Manderino and Berkey 1997). Some speculate that verbal abuse by physicians contributes significantly to horizontal hostility because nurses pass their anger and frustration with physicians onto vulnerable coworkers.

Nurses often cite verbal abuse from peers and supervisors as a reason for leaving their jobs. "Researchers report that verbal abuse contributes to 16%–24% of staff turnover and 25%–42% of nurse administrator turnover" (Braun et al. 1991; Cox 1991; Hilton et al. 1994). In the U.S., "the turnover rate is 33%–37% for clinical practicing nurses and 55%–61% for newly registered nurses. Approximately 60% of newly registered nurses leave their first position within six months because of some form of lateral violence" (Griffin 2004).

In addition, nurses who report the greatest degree of conflict with other nurses also report the highest rates of burnout (Hillhouse and Adler 1997). In 2001, Dr. Linda Aiken of the University of Pennsylvania's Center for Health Outcomes and Policy Research released a study that examined reports from 43,329 nurses from the United States, Canada, England, Scotland, and Germany. The study found that nurse dissatisfaction was high in all of those countries except for Germany. Burnout and dissatisfaction were reported by 43% of U.S. nurses, and 27.7% planned to leave the profession within a year (Aiken 2001). In a nursing shortage, these statistics are especially foreboding and demand that every nurse, on every level, accept the challenge of ending nurse-to-nurse hostility and creating a new culture.

Note that horizontal hostility is not limited to females. "We saw many instances of [horizontal hostility] in our sample of male RNs. They too made disparaging remarks about colleagues. They too experienced frequent verbal attacks by co-workers. One male nurse spoke of being 'wounded with words.' Another said, 'She purposely attacked me, embarrassing me in front of others, humiliating me, trying to make me look incompetent' "(Thomas 2003).

As a front-line manager, I have witnessed horizontal hostility on numerous occasions. One nurse would constantly write up other nurses, rather than speaking to those particular nurses directly. It was not unusual for me to come into the office in the morning and find three incident reports in my box written on the same person. Problems arose because new hires and resident nurses found it difficult to fit into a "clique." Comments like "I hate to follow *her*" were common. The longer the nurses had worked together, the harder it was for others to join their group. Nurses would constantly put down each other by making snide comments, and new nurses struggled to be perfect, knowing that every mistake would be seen as a direct reflection of their competence. Much to my chagrin, the practice of horizontal hostility was quite common on the unit.

Of all the types of aggression that nurses encounter (patient-to-nurse, nurse-to-visitor, doctor-to-nurse, and nurse-to-nurse), nurses report that the **most distressing type of aggression to deal with is nurse-to-nurse aggression** (Farrell 1999). Such intrapersonal conflicts rob us of our energy, deflect our interests from patient care, and prevent us from unifying in order to obtain the resources we need to do our jobs. The consequences of horizontal hostility can be felt on all levels: individual, professional, and organizational.

Impact

Individual impact

"In the societies of the highly industrialized western world, the workplace is the only remaining battlefield where people can 'kill' each other without running the risk of being taken to court."

—*Namie and Namie,* The Bully at Work

The effects of a hostile work environment cannot be minimized. Research shows that verbal abuse significantly affects the work environment by decreasing morale, increasing job dissatisfaction, and creating hostility (Manderino and Berkey 1997; Aiken 2001). Bullied staff report a decreased sense of relaxation and well-being at work, increased mistrust, low self-esteem, and lack of support from both staff and superiors (Cook et al. 2001).

Victims of horizontal hostility experience a wide range of emotional, social, psychological, and physical consequences. For example, the medical community recognizes several physical ailments as being triggered or aggravated by stress: irritable bowel syndrome, migraines, hypertension, allergies and asthma, arthritis, and fibromyalgia. Emotional-psychological damage can be less obvious and can include poor concentration and forgetfulness, loss of sleep or fatigue, indecisiveness, anxiety and nightmares, and obsessive thinking about a bully (Namie and Namie 2000).

At the October 2005 conference on horizontal violence, Gerald Farrell, RN, PhD, summarized some of the known effects of verbal abuse:

Emotional

- Anger, irritability
- Decreased self-esteem, self-doubt
- Lack of motivation and feelings of failure from being unable to meet personal expectations

Social

- Strained relationships with partner and friends (One-third to one-half of relationships between partners and family members worsen after someone *simply witnesses* bullying)
- Low interpersonal support/absence of emotional support

Psychological

- Depression
- PTSD—50% continue to suffer from stress five years after the incident
- Burnout—depersonalization, lack of control
- Maladaptive responses—substance abuse, overeating

Physical

- Decreased immune response or resistance to infection
- Cardiac arrhythmias (increased risk of heart attack due to continuously circulating catecholamines)

Seasoned nurses may recall that 20 years ago, new grads were treated as they often are today—harshly, as though they were being hazed to earn membership into the group. But many nurses do not remember horizontal hostility to the extent that it exists now. Little research documents when this behavior escalated and spread from new grads to staff nurses. Informal conversations seem to point to the late 1990s, when managed care and hospital mergers restructured the healthcare setting. At the time, no one realized the tremendous impact these changes would have on people (Weinberg 2003). The financial gains promised were never delivered because no one took into account the most critical factor of all—human factors. For example, feelings of identity were threatened, and feelings of fear and loss resulted in serious culture conflicts. During this time period, between two thirds and three fourths of all industries, including hospitals, failed to meet their predicted economic gains because the impact of mergers on culture was overlooked (Cartwright and Cooper 1993; Marks and Mirvis 1992). Culture, researchers have found, is critical.

Organizational impact

"It is imperative that healthcare organizations re-examine workplace concerns with the goal of creating environments that support nurses in their endeavors to provide quality care."

—*Sofield and Salmond (2003)*

Nothing is as destructive to an organization as a toxic work environment. Horizontal hostility creates such an environment by producing feelings of inferiority, anger, powerlessness, and frustration, which are counterproductive when working in a group. Emotional issues will incapacitate even the greatest of initiatives. Horizontal hostility "is a self-serving, non-productive response that perpetuates an escalating cycle of resentment and retaliation" (O'Hare and O'Hare 2004), and research shows that the interpersonal conflict it causes has a direct negative impact on intragroup conflict and work satisfaction (Cox 2003). Indeed, interpersonal conflicts affect teamwork, patient safety, and quality of care (Leppa 1996).

The emotional and physical health of employees is a product of the work environment and a key factor in group dynamics. When horizontal hostility enters the picture, it detrimentally affects the environment by producing a host of physical ailments that result in a loss of time from work (absenteeism, time off with worker's compensation, family medical leave of absences) and reduced productivity while at work. These responses affect not only the organization's bottom line but also the efficiency of the entire facility.

The invisible thread that weaves us together is the quality of our relationships. High-quality relationships are reflected in cohesiveness or solidarity—employees who are "all on the same page" and who function with a clear vision of the organization's goals. Researchers have also noted a direct link between high rates of group cohesion and work satisfaction and a lower turnover rate in acute care settings (Amos et al. 2005). Clearly, the "hallway conversations" that result from such cohesion often give us the critical information and support we need as we do our jobs. Now more then ever, streamlining processes and procedures in hospitals is critical to patient safety and financial efficiency.

The financial impact

"The effects of nursing stress have potentially enormous financial and human costs."
—*Hillhouse and Adler (1997)*

"Nursing leaders are becoming more aware of the costs and consequences of hostility among nurses to the healthcare system and to individual nurses" (Arle 2004). Some economic effects, such as high turnover rates, are obvious. Significant literature also validates the effects of stress and burnout on nurses (Aiken et al. 2002). For example, when positions need to be filled due to sick calls, compensation claims, and family medical leave of absences, overtime and agency costs accrue. An Australian study published in 1999 in the *Journal of Advanced Nursing* showed that 34% of nurses who experienced bullying took off more than 50 sick days in a year (Farrell 1999). In addition, the high cost of replacing nurses during a nursing shortage demands that we become aware of the reasons nurses are leaving.

Other economic costs are more difficult to quantify—e.g., the cost of decreased productivity as well as increased mistakes. In the same Australian study, 25% of nurses reported decreased productivity, and 27% reported impaired ability to perform their tasks. Studies confirm that verbal abuse causes a decrease in morale and an increase in errors and staff turnover.

Retention during a nursing shortage

As the nursing shortage becomes more critical, the reputation of hospitals and of specific units within those hospitals will become more important. Students in their clinical practicums will assess the quality of relationships and decide where they want to work based on their student experiences. Both new grads and floating inter-department nurses will choose to work on nursing units where they feel valued and supported, so creating a healthy work environment will give facilities a proven competitive advantage.

The nursing shortage projections are well documented and well known. According to the U.S. Bureau of Labor Statistics, more than one million new and replacement nurses will be needed by 2012. But even as we head toward the worst nursing shortage in history, the total number of RNs is growing at the slowest rate in 20 years, further compounding the problem. Forty percent of nursing schools are turning away students due to lack of faculty, and the mean nurse faculty age is 51 years old. Universities cannot compete with the high salaries that an advanced-prepared nurse can earn in the private sector, so the pool of nurses with master's and doctorate degrees will continue to decrease, resulting in a shortage of educators (American Association of Colleges of Nursing).

Ultimately, the shortage comes down to what each of us can control on our own level. As managers, directors, CNOs, and educators, we must make it a priority to learn why nurses are leaving our profession.

A root cause analysis performed after an episode of over-sedation revealed that the nurse was upset about an interaction with a coworker. Tearfully she stammered to the charge nurse, "I know I shouldn't have let [my coworker] get to me, but he did, and I just wasn't thinking clearly. I felt so humiliated, so belittled."

The nurse had inadvertently programmed the PCA to deliver 10 times the ordered dose of morphine. The patient was found unresponsive, with an oxygen saturation of 50%, and was transferred to the ICU. Two days later, a brain scan still showed areas of hypoxia, and the patient still could not put thoughts together clearly.

The nurse transferred to another department within the month. In her department exit interview, the nurse told the manager that she "had always wanted to work on the other unit and wanted to take advantage of the opportunity to transfer."

Summary

Of all types of aggression a nurse experiences, peer-to-peer hostility is the most hurtful (Farrell 1999). Studying this issue had been hampered by the lack of a universally accepted definition, as well as by a lack of awareness by staff nurses and leaders that the problem exists. Tales from the front line are consistent with the research and demonstrate the tremendous personal, professional, and organizational impact of this behavior.

Nurses who experience the highest degree of conflict also report the highest degree of burnout (Hillhouse and Adler 1997). The effects of a hostile environment are reflected in poor patient and employee satisfaction scores and, ultimately, in the reputation of the hospital or academic setting. New nurses will be drawn to healthy environments; it is therefore imperative that we acknowledge that horizontal hostility is a serious problem and learn strategies to intervene.

Recommended reading

Social Intelligence
    By Daniel Goleman

Bibliography

Adams, A. 1997. *Bullying at work—how to confront and overcome it.* London: Virago Press.

Aiken, L. et al. 2001. Nurses' reports on hospital care in five countries. *Health Affairs* 20(3): 43–53.

Aiken, L. et al. 2002. Hospital Nurse Staffing and Patient Mortality, Nurse Burnout, and Job Dissatisfaction. *Journal of the American Medical Association* 288: 1987–1993.

American Association of Colleges of Nursing. Nursing Shortage Fact Sheet. *www.aacn.nche.edu/Media/shortageresource.htm.*

Amos, M., H. Hu, and C. Herrick. 2005. The impact of team building on communication and job satisfaction of nursing staff. *Journal for Nurses in Staff Development* 21(1).

Arle, L. 2004. Horizontal caring in nursing and a narrative community experience. Unpublished thesis for Masters in Nursing. Washington State University, Washington.

Braun, K., et al. 1991. Verbal abuse of nurses and non-nurses. *Nursing Management* 22(30): 72–76.

Buback, D. 2004. Home Study Program: Assertiveness training to prevent verbal abuse in the OR. *AORN Journal* 79(1): 148–164.

Cartwright, S., and C. Cooper. 1993. The psychological impact of merger and acquisition on the individual: A study of building society managers. *Human Relations* 46(3): 327–348.

Cook, J. et al. 2001. Exploring the impact of physician verbal abuse on perioperative nurses. *AORN Journal* 74(3): 317–330.

Cox, H. 1991. Verbal abuse nationwide, Part II: Impact and modifications. *Nursing Management* 22(3): 66–69.

Cox, K. 2003. The Effects of Intrapersonal, Intragroup, and Intergroup Conflict on Team Performance Effectiveness and Work Satisfaction. *Nursing Administration Quarterly,* 27(2).

Dunn, H. 2003. Horizontal violence among nurses in the operating room. *AORN Journal* 78(6).

Farrell, G. 1999. Aggression in clinical settings: nurses' views—a follow-up study. *Journal of Advanced Nursing* 29(3): 532–541.

Farrell, G. 2005. "Issues in Nursing: Violence in the Workplace" conference. Tualatin, Oregon. Sponsored by the Oregon Chapter of the American Psychiatric Nurses Association.

Gilmour, D., and L. Hamlin. 2003. Bullying and harassment in perioperative settings. *British Journal of Perioperative Nursing* 13(2): 79–85.

Griffin, M, 2004. Teaching cognitive rehearsal as a shield for lateral violence: an intervention for newly licensed nurses. *The Journal of Continuing Education in Nursing* 35(6).

Hillhouse, J., and C. Adler. 1997. Investigating stress effect patterns in hospital staff nurses: results of a cluster analysis. *Social Science and Medicine* 45(12): 1781–1788.

Hilton, P., J. Kottke and D. Pfahler. 1994. Verbal abuse in nursing: How serious is it? *Nursing Management* 25(5): 90.

Leppa, C. 1996. Nurse relationships and work group disruption. *Journal of Nursing Administration* 26(10): 23–27.

Manderino, M., and N. Berkey. 1997. Verbal abuse of staff nurses by physicians. *Journal of Professional Nursing* 13(1): 48–55.

Marks, M., and P. Mirvis. 1992. Rebuilding after the merger: Dealing with survivor sickness. *Organizational Dynamics* 21(2):18–33.

McMillan, I. 1995. Losing control. *Nursing Times* 91(15): 40–43.

Namie, G., and R. Namie. 2000. *The Bully at Work: What You Can Do to Stop the Hurt and Reclaim Your Dignity on the Job.* Naperville, IL: Sourcebooks, Inc.

O'Hare, M., and J. O'Hare. 2004. Don't perpetuate horizontal violence. *Nursing Spectrum.*

Quine, L. 1999. Workplace bullying in NHS community trust: Staff questionnaire survey. *British Medical Journal* 318: 228–232.

Sofield, L., and S. Salmond. 2003. Workplace Violence: A Focus on Verbal Abuse and Intent to Leave the Organization. *Orthopaedic Nursing* 22(4): 274–283.

Thomas, S. 2003. "Horizontal Hostility": Nurses against themselves: How to resolve this threat to retention. *Journal of Advanced Nursing* 103(10).

Weinberg, D. 2003. *Code green: Money driven hospitals and the dismantling of nursing.* Ithaca, NY: Cornell University Press.

Exploring theory

Marie's story: A manager's point of view

Quitting was heart-wrenching. As I turned the key to lock my office door for the very last time, a thought occurred to me: I was doomed from the first time I ever opened this door. I never had a chance—and I never saw it coming.

It had taken me almost six months to quit because something I just couldn't quite put my finger on was holding me back. I remembered the advice of a wise friend who had said, "You can't close one door and open another until all the lessons have been learned." For months, I had struggled to understand what else I could possibly learn from this job. After seven years working 60+ hours every week managing a large surgical unit, I was frustrated and exhausted. I felt like 90% of my energy was spent just trying to get the resources I needed to do the job "they" expected. Articulating my unit's needs felt like screaming into an echoing abyss. I hadn't exercised in two years and was suffering from every classic symptom of burnout. So why, then, was it so difficult to quit? What was wrong with me?

Then one day, when I was getting onto the elevator, I simply "got it." I looked at another manager who was already in the elevator and, as we said our perfunctory hellos, a sickening feeling punched me in the gut. As always, her eyes were riveted to the floor in order to avoid any chance of conversation. Suddenly I remembered a book that I had read a long time ago, Clan of the Cave Bear. *In the story, the cave man society decides that Ayla does not exist. No matter how frantically Ayla waves her hands in front of their faces or clutches for her mother's hand, the tribe ignores her. It was society's worst form of punishment because members would die from being ignored.*

I looked at the manager's dispassionate face and saw what I feared: I was dying of loneliness. Despite having good relationships with my staff, physicians, and administration, I had been banned by my peers, but I hadn't the faintest idea why. The years of being ignored were taking their toll.

At this point, all I really knew was how I felt. Suddenly, I remembered a story my teacher had told me about Romanian orphans in the 1950s. Hundreds of infants were routinely diapered and their bottles propped up in their cribs, but so many babies were dying that the government sent for a team from the United States to help determine the cause of death. The infants, they discovered, were dying because of lack of touch. And so, before the elevator doors even opened again, I saw myself reaching out through the bars, dying from rejection, from invisibility, due to lack of human touch. The depth of the rejection was the lesson that had been too painful to acknowledge.

I went back to my office with the realization that I could never move into another position at this institution because I was not supported by with my peers. I had received absolutely no training, and even if I had, it wouldn't have mattered—I didn't learn the rules until too late in the game. And so I quit. I felt so torn. I really loved my staff.

Oppression theory

"Oppression elicits negative behaviors: silence, a lack of voice, poor self-esteem, and the sublimation of the experience of powerlessness through the internal divisiveness known as horizontal violence."

—Demarco et al. (2005)

The term horizontal violence was first coined by theorist Paulo Freire in 1972 to explain the conflict that existed in colonized African populations. Freire observed that an imbalance of power always resulted in the formation of a dominant and a subordinate group. Whenever there are two groups and one has more power than the other, he argued, oppression occurs when the values of the subordinate culture are repressed. This is called the oppression theory.

Freire noted that the subordinate group would feel inferior because they were forced to reject their own values and characteristics in order to maintain the status quo. As members of the subordinate group acted out their feelings of self-hatred on one another, internal conflict began to spread. The values, beliefs, and characteristics that the Africans had once respected and cherished in themselves were lost.

In 1983, Sandra Roberts, PhD, RN, FAAN, applied oppression theory to nursing and argued that "an understanding of the dynamics underlying leadership of an oppressed group is important if strategy to develop more effective leaders in nursing is to be successful" (1983). She noted that nursing displayed many of the characteristics of an oppressed group: low self-esteem, self-hatred, and feelings of powerlessness.

Founded in a patriarchal society and composed predominately of women, the nursing profession was set up from the start to assume a subordinate position. It is not hard to imagine the circumstances under which the nursing profession originated: In a time when women had practically no rights, nursing provided women with an opportunity to escape their fate and stand on their own. Yet in order for this new profession to be acceptable—especially given that the women would be caring for men who were strangers—nursing was portrayed as a "calling," or as "God's work" (Reverby 1987). Nurses were viewed as angels of mercy—and angels don't get angry.

From this new paradigm came a set of expectations, albeit unrealistic, that nurses struggled to meet:

- A nurse is consistently caring.
- A nurse rejects her own needs and works long hours for little reward.
- A nurse never complains.
- A nurse is always subordinate and speaks only when spoken to.

Significant literature substantiates the idea that nursing is an oppressed discipline (Roberts 1983; David 2000; Torres 1981) and that the origins of this oppression can be traced back to gender issues (Kanter 1979; Farrell 1997; Reverby 1987; Gordon 2005). Hence, nursing is "an oppression by gender and an oppression by medical dominance" (Dargon 1999), with physicians often assuming dominance over their "subordinates."

Any profession that holds a belief system rooted in subordination will feel oppressed, and horizontal hostility is the natural expression of this suppressed anger. Add to the equation the increased pressures incurred by nurses after the

restructuring of healthcare in the 1990s (which resulted in a hierarchical organizational structure with little nursing representation), and it is easy to see how
horizontal hostility has gained momentum.

The culture of oppression in nursing

Debby is complaining again. As I walk onto the floor, the air hangs in her negativity.

*"What's the problem, Debby?" I say to her and to the group of nurses all huddled
around the main station.*

*It takes me several minutes to drag it out of her. The problem, it seems, is that a new
nurse is not working weekends, and Debby is resentful.*

*"Debby, we have had self-scheduling for more than two years now. If you don't want to
work weekends, just change the schedule." She looks at me in shock.*

*"What do you mean?" she asks, her voice filled with disbelief. "Do you mean that for
two years now I could have had off every single weekend?"*

"Yes."

*Debby does not make a dash for the schedule but instead stands there, flabbergasted,
trying to comprehend how or why she did not understand that the prison door was never
locked; she could have walked out any time.*

Now it is my turn to take in what happens to people when they work in the nursing culture for a long time. The term "learned helplessness" takes on special meaning. Oppression is no longer a buzz word from my theory class.

One of the defining features of oppression is that both the dominant and the subordinate groups internalize the norms set by the dominant group and accept them as normal. After a period of time, no one—not even the subordinate group—notices or questions these unspoken rules (Roberts 1983). This pattern occurs today in the behaviors of physicians and nurses. Nurses are not aware of how the dominating actions of physicians—such as avoiding direct eye contact, not bothering to learn a nurse's name, and having only abrupt conversations— keep nurses in the subordinate position (Bartholomew 2004). What, then, are the behaviors of *nurses* that we do not see, that we accept as normal, and that perpetuate horizontal hostility? One is that new nurses accept the culture they walk into as "normal." As one new nurse said to me, "I was never a nurse before. I thought it was normal for the new nurse to answer call lights for 18 patients while the experienced nurse sat and knitted."

Horizontal hostility is often accepted as "normal" and is, in my experience, not consciously committed by the perpetrator. One theoretical explanation for this is suppression, which "occurs when thoughts and emotions are either consciously or unconsciously eliminated from awareness. In this way, the individual is protected from overwhelming anxiety or helplessness" (Farrell 2001). The nurse may not be conscious of the harm she is causing if she is responding to oppression of which she is not aware.

Powerlessness

When anger is suppressed and cannot be directed upward, nurses lash out against each other.

There had always been a lot of tension between another manager and myself, so I thought it might helpful to explain the oppression model to her. When I said that we were an oppressed group and that the backstabbing and low self-esteem we suffered were related to our powerlessness, Margaret vehemently disagreed.

"Do you feel like you have power?" I asked.

"Why, yes," she responded.

I tried to recall some specific examples. "Remember when the budget was due and if any manager needed more hours of care, we had to take them from another manager because there was only a fixed number of FTEs? It was like a scene from Oliver Twist! There we were, all starving for hours of care, and whoever wanted more had to beg from someone else who was already understaffed!"

Margaret still wasn't convinced. I thought of another example. "We are supposed to round with staff frequently, asking whether they have what they need to do their jobs, but no one would ever dream of ever asking us! Do you have what you need to do YOUR job?"

End of conversation. Margaret stood up and walked away—either she couldn't see the truth or didn't want to.

Our perception of our own powerlessness is the root cause of horizontal hostility, yet the powerlessness itself is so ingrained that we do not acknowledge its role in the social construct of nursing. This invisibility may be closely tied to gender definitions. Power is rejected (on a subconscious level) by the subordinate group because it is viewed as a dominant group characteristic. "Traditional conceptualization of power and caring are presented as polar opposites . . . power is congruent with the characteristics of masculinity, whereas the characteristics of femininity prepare women to care" (Falk-Rafael 1996).

In the oppression model, the values of the subordinate group—in this case, caring—are denigrated by the dominant group and, at the same time, the values of the dominant group—in this case, power—are elevated. Unconsciously, the subordinate group pushes away its own values because they are perceived as a dominant group characteristic. The subordinate group, therefore, is left powerless and with a weakened sense of self. Such an extreme power differential between the subordinate group and the dominant group creates an undertow whose strength we do not see, and it takes the nursing profession far off-course. Margaret has no idea where she is.

The purpose of the "veil of oppression," as Roberts refers to it, is to prevent us from seeing the truth (1983). This veil is thin enough to see through, yet we do not acknowledge its presence or take it off because we don't even realize it's there. The veil keeps us hidden. *Why is being invisible so important to nurses?*

Invisibility

Five years of being ignored went by, and then one day I finally heard the gossip about me. "Who does she think she is, having a three-day retreat for her charge nurses? Where did she get the money?"

Then one day a peer stopped me in the hall after I had obtained a much needed 0.5 support position and caught me totally off-guard. "You better be quiet now, missy. Now that you got what you wanted, you had better just keep that mouth of yours shut."

Herein lies the Catch 22: At a very primal level, there is an unspoken belief that nursing's identity must stay invisible in order to survive. **Yet it is this very invisibility that keeps the group in the subordinate, oppressed position and prevents solidarity.** "Infighting within the profession prevents mobilization of resources to confront the larger issues of healthcare reform" (Smith et al. 1996).

The current system keeps nurses invisible and subordinate. In her book, *Nursing Against the Odds*, Suzanne Gordon expertly identifies how this invisibility is kept alive—from physicians taking credit for nurses' work to daily failures to acknowledge nurses' contributions. Such a structure causes problems: "Years of invisibility take their toll. When nurses get no positive public credit for their work, [their] sense of professional self-worth slowly erodes" (Gordon 2005). In addition, when nurses cannot practice from within their value set, their self-esteem falters. For example, caring—a cherished value—has assumed a position of little importance in today's traditional hierarchical institution; it is difficult to quantify, and even harder to fit into the budget. As a result, nurses feel insignificant and undervalued.

The organizational hierarchy also invalidates another nursing value: the concept of reflection. In a study published in 2004 in the *Journal of Clinical Nursing*, researchers found that nurses who participated in reflective practice were made to feel that they were outside the norm (Mantzoukas and Jasper 2004). Yet reflective practice is a key mechanism in understanding and processing our nursing experiences.

The oppression model thus offers a reasonable explanation for many other theories put forth to explain horizontal hostility, including hierarchical abuse, clique formation, low self-esteem, and the inadequate response of nurse managers. Under this model, hierarchical abuse is an effort of the dominant group to keep the subordinate group in their place. Clique formation is a survival mechanism—people band together to weather the stress of oppression. Low self-esteem, a known characteristic of any oppressed group, stems from a rejection of core values. And the inadequate response from nurse managers (in dealing with horizontal hostility) occurs because they have taken on the characteristics of the dominant group.

Weakened sense of identity

"I spend all of this time filling out ten pages of a progress record and not once have I ever seen a physician even look at my charting. After working on the unit for 15 years, I think there's only one doctor who even knows my name."

Our invisibility is a significant contributor to our weak sense of identity. "Evidence that nursing is little known and misunderstood is all around us" (Buresh and Gordon 2003). In the controversial case of Terri Schiavo, the nurses who took care of Terri were noticeably absent from media discussion, even though they had cared for her for years. Nurses are not among expert sources quoted in news stories or analyses of mistakes in healthcare (Buresh and Gordon 2003). Although nursing is the largest profession in healthcare, it is also the quietest—from an organizational standpoint, down to each individual nurse. As was true for the colonized Africans in Freire's study, the cultural identity of nurses has suffered. The skill and art of nursing have progressively lost value as technology and science assume a greater level of importance in our society. Organizational restructuring has removed nurses from key decision-making positions. Without a voice and without representation, nursing has slowly fallen by the wayside.

Supporting theory: Insights from the animal kingdom

Psychological stress and displaced aggression

If a rat is subjected to a stressor such as a series of very mild shocks, he develops a prolonged stress response—his glucocorticoid levels increase, as does his probability of developing an ulcer. However, if the rat is given a block of wood to run over and chew on when the stress occurs, he is far less likely to get an ulcer because he has an outlet for his frustration. If a rat receives a mild shock and there is another rat in the cage, he will "run over, sit next to the rat [and] bite the hell out of it" (Sapolsky 1998). **Scientists refer to this as "stress-induced displacement aggression." Nurses refer to it as "eating their young."**

Two other important factors identified in the rat stress studies were predictability and the perception of control over a situation. Whereas unpredictability increased the stress response, *just the perception of control* over a stressor decreased its effect. In nursing, we lose out on all three counts; we do not have an outlet for our frustration, unpredictability is high, and the perception that we have control is low.

Psychological stress and social support

Primates also exhibit a great deal of displaced aggression. If a male baboon loses a fight, he will turn around and attack a baboon who was just sitting there minding his own business. But scientists have also noticed something else about the primates' stress response: Given the exact same stressor, "the primates react differently *depending on who is in the room*" (Sapolsky 1998). If the others present are strangers, then the stress is worse. If the primate's friends are in the room, then the stress response decreases. Social support networks, therefore, significantly affect how primates handle psychological stress. "Profound and persistent differences in degrees of social support can influence human physiology as well" (Sapolsky 1998).

The implications for nursing are clear: In the drive for increased efficiency and productivity, opportunities for social support have decreased significantly—especially after the creation of 12-hour shifts. The impact of low social support at work is compounded by the fact that social capital—the time we have to connect with each other—has decreased tremendously in our society (Putnam 2000). Our social support networks at work and at home are clearly lacking, which contributes to an increase in our psychological stress.

Populations at risk

"Bullies scan groups for the weakest. Maybe it is an evolutionary remnant of our place in the animal kingdom. All predatory species select and attack the weakest prey."
—*Namie and Namie,* The Bully at Work

Whether a new hire, a transfer from another department, or a new resident nurse, any member introduced into a powerless group is at high risk for experiencing horizontal hostility. Horizontal hostility is used to break new nurses into the group or, in terms of oppression theory, to acculturate them into the group. This is how we teach those unspoken rules. If the status quo is rocked in any way, fear escalates and expresses itself as horizontal hostility. It's as if "until she is one of us, she is a threat." The last thing new nurses need today, however, is a difficult rite of passage.

While new graduates are easy prey to horizontal hostility, nurse managers are also extremely vulnerable targets due to their marginalization and relative isolation from each other. In other words, nurse managers do not typically feel at ease eating lunch with the staff nurses they supervise or the administration to whom they answer. Therefore, this group has a particularly weak identity unless championed by a strong nursing administration and given the time necessary to build solid relationships.

Marginalized groups tend to take on the characteristics of the dominant group. This pattern might explain the comments staff nurses make about new nurse managers, such as, "She is always in her office doing paperwork," "She's one of *them* now," or, "She has no clue what is going on in the floor because we never see her."

Managers or staff members are especially vulnerable if they act differently than other members of the group because their behavior inadvertently draws attention and threatens the group's invisibility. Like the child of an alcoholic parent, a nurse sees his or her invisibility as a means of staying out of harm's way and out of the spotlight. Unnecessary attention puts the entire group in danger—it doesn't matter if this attention is for the good of the group. Thus, a manager who excels, complains, dresses differently, etc., is immediately perceived as a threat *at the most primal level* because she is standing up to the dominant group. Her actions run the risk of retaliation by the dominant group against the entire subordinate group. To prevent this from happening, the subordinate group immediately demonstrates behaviors that will cause that nurse to leave the group. Gossiping, backstabbing, ignoring, etc., are all means toward this end. These behaviors, designed to extricate the nurse from the group, are unconsciously considered vital to the survival of the group.

"You wouldn't think it would happen to a director, but they ran her out. They sabotaged her and ignored her until she quit. That one only lasted a year. I could see how they distanced themselves from her. She always sat alone."

Figure 2.1	The 10 most frequent forms of lateral violence in nursing practice*

1. Nonverbal innuendo (raising of eyebrows, face-making)
2. Verbal affront (covert or overt, snide remarks, lack of openness, abrupt responses)
3. Undermining activities (turning away, not available)
4. Withholding information (practice or patient)
5. Sabotage (deliberately setting up a negative situation)
6. Infighting (bickering with peers)
7. Scapegoating (attributing all that goes wrong to one individual)
8. Backstabbing (complaining to others about an individual and not speaking directly to that individual)
9. Failure to respect privacy
10. Broken confidences

* Ordered from most to least frequently encountered.
Adapted from Duffy, 1995; Farrell, 1997; McCall, 1996; McKenna, Smith, Poole, & Coverdale, 2003. SLACK Incorporated and The Journal of Continuing Education in Nursing. *Reprinted with permission.*

Why is horizontal hostility so virulent?

Denial

The strongest force that perpetuates horizontal hostility is denial—denial by both the nurses who are committing the hostile behaviors *and* the targets who are keeping silent. When any behavior has been a part of a culture for a very long time, it is perceived as normal.

Witnesses also play a role in perpetuating horizontal hostility. For example, senior nurses witness overt behaviors intended to diminish new nurses on the unit; what they see matches their own orientation, so they don't identify the behaviors as a problem. All the players in this drama—the victim, the perpetrator, and the witness—fail to acknowledge the problem or take any action.

Hostility's visibility

In addition to hostility being accepted as the norm, hospital restructuring has significantly increased the manager's scope of practice, making these key individuals less visible than ever before.

"I had four units! There was supposed to be a supervisor in each of those units, but a year went by and no one had applied for the position in three of the units. So there I was trying to get the schedules out for 300 people. It was insane. I worked 12–14 hours a day and weekends."

This increased workload has significantly decreased the manager's presence on the unit, as managers struggle with the paperwork (incident reports, budgets, schedules, position requisitions, etc.) for multiple units. The system was not set up to support the manager. Thus, hostility has become even less visible to the only person with the power and authority to interrupt it. The manager is now noticeably absent.

Ineffective supervisor intervention

"She was like gangrene. I told the director that she was infecting all of us, but still she [the director] did nothing. I told her again and again. Finally, people started leaving, and there was a mass exodus. She just wouldn't cut her off so that we could all live."

Managers have been accused of not responding appropriately to staff concerns about horizontal hostility. "Nurse managers are blamed more for acts of omission than for acts of commission" (Farrell 2001). Many nurses who complain to their managers do not feel like it makes any difference (Farrell 2005). Managers may fail to respond for several reasons: their assimilation into the dominant group, a heavy workload, poor conflict management skills, inadequate education/role modeling, feelings of helplessness (or lack of support), and an underlying perception that hostility is the norm. In a study conducted by Gerald Farrell, PhD, RN, for his PhD dissertation at the University of Tasmania, Australia, Farrell found that respondents' main concern about nurse managers was "their failure to implement supportive structures when incidents arose or to take appropriate action to prevent their reoccurrence" (2001).

Lack of confrontation skills

I asked the charge nurse to come into my office with the staff nurse at the end of the day because they were both so angry and upset with each other. Suddenly, the charge nurse started to cry and quickly covered her eyes with her hands.

"Would you like to do this at another time?" I asked.

"No," she responded, "I'll be okay. Just give me a minute. It's just my alcoholic father—stuff from childhood," she said, composing herself again. "Go on . . ."

Nurses frequently demonstrate a passive-aggressive communication style; some speculate that this is due to childhood experiences in which one parent abused a substance. From childhood, they bring the message that "Herculean measures should be attempted rather than ever rocking the boat." Maintaining the status quo becomes equivalent to avoiding conflict at all costs. The innate desire to care for others may have also emerged from these childhood experiences—used to "taking care" of things at home, they were drawn to nursing as a profession.

Thus, charge nurses who have been on the unit for many years may lack leadership skills—specifically, confrontation/conflict management skills—because of the passivity they developed in childhood. And without supervisory constraints in place, horizontal hostility goes unchecked. Staff continue their behavior without any consequence.

Professional denial

It is hard to admit that we who chose the nursing profession could be so mean to each other. The foundation of our work is caring. But as pointed out earlier, caring is not a value honored by the dominant group. It has been diminished in the power struggle that exists wherever there is a hierarchy. Working in an environment that does not honor caring lowers our self-esteem and creates a great deal of moral dissatisfaction—and this unhappiness triggers hostility.

Intermittent reinforcement: Aggression breeds aggression

One of the critical forces keeping horizontal hostility in motion is intermittent reinforcement (Farrell 2005). Skinner discovered that the strongest way to reinforce a behavior was not continuous reinforcement, but rather *intermittent* reinforcement. Sporadic and surprise verbal attacks thus create a hyper-vigilance—if one does not know when hostility will strike, one will always be on guard.

Being abused is a vicious cycle that leads to increased levels of hostility. That is, "once aggression arises, it is likely to be maintained unless remedial action is taken" (Farrell 1999).

Pressure relief

When we "vent," we release pressure. Over the past decade there has been a tremendous increase in the pressures felt by the nurse. The human adaptability theory, which states that incremental increases in pressure over time go unrecognized, allows pressure to build up without notice.

Pressure comes from the fact that length of stay has decreased, patient acuity has increased, the weight of patients has increased, and the average age of nurses has increased. Nurses may reluctantly admit that they "were blowing off steam" when they acted out against a coworker.

A nurse who had worked on our unit several years before returned to apply for an evening position. Before interviewing her, I gathered some information from staff who had worked with her in the past. "Is she a good nurse?" I asked.

The nurses responded that, yes, she was clinically sound, but that she was "extremely negative." They did not want to experience her negativity again.

During the interview process I relayed the acceptable and unacceptable behaviors on our unit, when suddenly she interrupted me.

"Wait," she said emphatically. "It's only natural for a nurse to vent; it's a part of the job. When you are frustrated, you have to let it out."

"No," I responded, "that is not our culture here. If you are frustrated on our floor, you have two options:
1. Talk directly to the person you are frustrated with in private, or
2. Come and talk to me."

I was not surprised when she withdrew her application a week later.

Summary

The nursing group will never elevate itself from the subordinate position as long as it is invisible. And the only way to become visible is to
- Lift the veil of oppression. Nursing leaders must acknowledge the oppression and powerlessness and illuminate the hostility.
- Elevate the self-esteem of nurses individually and collectively (Roberts 1983).

The oppression model provides a working conceptual framework for understanding horizontal hostility in nursing. It not only explains *why* horizontal hostility exists but, more importantly, holds the key to breaking this vicious cycle of aggression.

On a very practical level, the key is to

- hold staff accountable for hostile behaviors
- insist upon a crucial conversation between both parties when any nurse experiences hostility

Time and time again my experience has shown me that the behaviors stop as soon as the perpetrators comprehend the damage they are causing. It is the very understanding of these dynamics that will result in nurses reclaiming their power.

Bibliography

Bartholomew, K. 2004. *Speak Your Truth: Proven Strategies for Effective Nurse-Physician Communication.* Marblehead, MA: HCPro, Inc.

Buresh, B., and S. Gordon. 2003. *From Silence to Voice: What nurses know and must communicate to the public.* Ithaca, NY: Cornell University Press.

Dargon, M. 1999. Disrupting oppression theory. Unpublished thesis for Masters in Nursing. University of Tasmania, Launceston, Australia.

David, B. 2000. Nursing's gender politics; reformulating the footnotes. *Advances in Nursing Science,* 23(1): 83–93.

DeMarco, R., S. Roberts, and G. Chandler. 2005. The use of a writing group to enhance voice and connection among staff nurses. *Journal for Nurses in Staff Development* 21(3): 85–90.

Falk-Rafael, A. 1996. Power and caring: A dialectic in nursing. *Advances in Nursing Science* 19(1): 3–17.

Farrell, G. 1997. Aggression in clinical settings: Nurses' views. *Journal of Advanced Nursing* 25: 501–508.

Farrell, G. 1999. Aggression in clinical settings: Nurses' views—a follow-up study. *Journal of Advanced Nursing* 29(3): 532–541.

Farrell, G. 2001. From tall poppies to squashed weeds: Why don't nurses pull together more? *Journal of Advanced Nursing* 35(1): 26–33.

Farrell, G. 2005. "Issues in Nursing: Violence in the Workplace" conference. Tualatin, Oregon. Sponsored by the Oregon Chapter of the American Psychiatric Nurses Association.

Freire, P. 1990. *Pedagogy of the Oppressed.* New York: Continuum International Publishing Group.

Gordon, S. 2005. *Nursing Against the Odds: How Health Care Cost Cutting, Media Stereotypes, and Medical Hubris Undermine Nurses and Patient Care (The Culture and Politics of Healthcare Work).* Ithaca, NY: ILR Press.

Kanter, R. 1979. Power failure in management circuits. *Harvard Business Review* 57(4): 65–75.

Mantzoukas, S., and M. Jasper. 2004. Reflective practice and daily ward reality: a covert power game. *Journal of Clinical Nursing* 13(8): 925–933.

Namie, G., and R. Namie. 2000. *The Bully at Work: What You Can Do to Stop the Hurt and Reclaim Your Dignity on the Job.* Naperville, IL: Sourcebooks, Inc.

Putnam, R. 2000. *Bowling Alone: The collapse and revival of American community.* New York: Simon & Schuster.

Reverby, S. 1987. *Ordered to care: The dilemma of American nursing 1850–1945.* New York: Cambridge University Press.

Roberts, S. 1983 Oppressed group behavior: Implications for nursing. *Advances In Nursing Science* 5(4): 21–30.

Sapolsky, R. 1998. **Why** *Zebras Don't Get Ulcers: An updated guide to stress, stress-related diseases and coping.* New York: Freeman & Company.

Smith, M., P. Droppleman, and S. Thomas. 1996. Under assault: The experience of work-related anger in female registered nurses. *Nursing Forum* 31(1): 22–33.

Torres, G. 1981. The Nursing Education Administrator: Accountable, vulnerable and oppressed. *Advances in Nursing Science* 3: 1–16.

A root cause analysis of horizontal hostility

Marie's search for answers

A new administrator arrived at the hospital, and when she heard a piece of gossip, she immediately called me to her office. The current rumor was that I knew some "insider information" about a restructuring process and that I wanted my position posted as soon as possible. Neither was true.

"Then why the misinformation?" she asked. My heart fell. "It's the culture," I replied sadly, wondering if she would believe me. I didn't even want to believe me! But I couldn't find any other reason or pretend everything was okay any longer. The administrator encouraged me to find out how the gossip began.

I immediately called the manager who had started the gossip and arranged to go up to her office. Clearly upset, I told her what had just happened. Then, for the first time, I got to hear the gossip that had been circulating about me for seven years. I so appreciated her candor and her willingness to share. But why didn't anyone check things out? Why did no one talk to me—for seven years?

During our conversation, the manager would recall a past situation and relay the gossip, and then I would explain what had really happened. As soon as she saw my pain, she saw the truth. It was a powerful and emotional confrontation that ended with her promising "to stop the talking."

I could not hold back the tears as I walked out of her office. I felt transported back to the sixth-grade lunchroom. The work we were both doing was so very, very hard, and this whole time we could have been supporting each other—as if the challenges of healthcare were not enough! It felt like I had found a cure for a disease that had already killed me. It was too late—I had already given my notice. Even crucial conversations with all of my peers could not erase seven years of backstabbing. I felt defeated. I felt cheated.

Through exit interviews and conversations with administration, I managed to better understand my situation before my last day (I was lucky, for many nurses leave feeling incomprehensible alienation). Inadvertently, I had discovered the unspoken behavioral expectations inherent in the nursing culture. But it took me a long time to not take the rejection personally—I beat myself up about it for months. I try to tell myself that our group was just trying to survive, but some days it takes more convincing than others.

Marie's look back: A reflection interview

What did you mean by "I never had a chance" and "I never saw it coming"?

Marie: People who had been there for years had the power to smear you and did so before you even knew it was happening. It's like walking into a very important game where the stakes are really high (i.e., my job and feeding my kids), and the people you are playing with won't let you see the rule book. I hadn't realized nursing was so competitive. Lots of poker faces.

What did you learn in your exit interviews that was helpful?

Marie: That there was a piece of truth in this situation for me, too. I realized that I had never felt supported in my life and that I probably was projecting that to others. When I got past the pain, I was able to acknowledge the support I did receive from lots of other departments—just not nursing.

I stopped beating myself up because [other nurses] wouldn't let me in. I learned that it was only partly my responsibility to leverage myself with my peers—nursing administration had a responsibility to stop the gossip, but they let it continue, even when they knew it wasn't true. They didn't seem to recognize it for what it was. Nor were they aware of the damage.

I learned that my expectations were unrealistic and that a lot of my frustration had come from trying to work too hard to get the resources I needed. I should have monitored my energy better. At first, I didn't realize the constraints of working in a healthcare institution. Then I wholeheartedly believed that things would get better—and later, I couldn't accept that they didn't.

What were the rules that you didn't know but wish you had?

Marie: Don't do anything to set yourself apart.

> *Don't rock the boat in any way. Silence is golden.*
>
> *Don't trust ANYONE, ever. NEVER let your guard down.*
>
> *Never talk to anyone higher than your boss.*
>
> *If someone has a problem with you, you will never know it—but everyone else will.*
>
> *If you can't join the clique, you won't survive.*

Individual context

After I read Marie's story to a university professor, she responded, "I feel that way too. I try to connect with my peers, but everyone is so busy. The one meeting I do have each week with a colleague is strictly business—there's really no connecting on any meaningful level."

Together we reflected on the pressures that come not just from the university, institution, and nursing unit, but from all directions. In addition to stress generated by conflict with peers, nurses bring a host of extrinsic factors into the situation: the damage caused by poor physician-nurse relationships, disenfranchising work practices, and an increasing demand for higher productivity.

Looking at ourselves and identifying some of the intrinsic factors that foster our isolation and alienation—inadequate conflict management and communication skills, a belief system that does not match reality, a Type A personality, unmet expectations, and burnout—is a good place to start. Because horizontal hostility is a complex subject, understanding all of these perspectives will give nursing leaders the information they need to find solutions.

Intrinsic factors

- Emotional state—anger, burnout
- Personality style
- Beliefs and expectations
- Inadequate communication and conflict management skills

Our emotional state

"All too often we leave the workplace bone tired and soul weary, trying to shake off the sticky residue of moral distress, that awful realization that we could not give patients the care they deserved."

—*Thomas (2004)*

Anger

Our anger is an expression of our pain. It "is not channeled into constructive actions. It eats away at us inside and takes its toll. It spills over to our own peers, corroding relationships" (Thomas 2004).

"Jackie had been mad for weeks, but no one quite knew why. She just kept writing up people and pointing out omissions in charting. Some staff jokingly referred to her as 'the charting Nazi.' It got to the point that nurses evaded her constantly, and then overtime increased as nurses took more time with their charting in order to not be 'punished' by being written up."

Sandra P. Thomas, PhD, RN, FAAN, professor and director of the PhD Program in Nursing at the University of Tennessee in Knoxville, has studied women's anger for more than 15 years and has conducted studies with both men and women in nursing for more than a decade. In her research, Thomas found that women's anger involved a confusing mixture of feelings. She discovered that when women turn their anger inward, they feel helpless and powerless. However, when women *externalize* their anger they *still feel powerless* because they view an outburst as a lack of control (2004).

What precipitates this anger?

- Unfair or disrespectful treatment
- A lack of reciprocity in relationships (Thomas 2004)

We pay a high price for this anger: fatigue, physical health problems (cancer, obesity, and heart disease), depression, and substance abuse. We must stop the harm we are causing to ourselves and learn how to transform our anger into productive energy that will improve our working relationships—and our own well-being.

A recent study of 843 direct care hospital nurses found that nurses under 30 years of age were more likely to experience feelings of agitation, and less likely to employ techniques to manage their feelings. The authors recommend that experienced nurses serve as emotional mentors and that we recognize the emotional demands inherent in our work. Understanding the emotional work of nursing is a key factor in understanding burnout. (Erickson).

Burnout

"Forty percent of hospital nurses have burnout levels that exceed the norms for healthcare workers, and job dissatisfaction among hospital nurses is four times greater than the average for all U.S. workers" (Aiken et al. 2002).

In his book, *Overcoming Secondary Stress in Medical and Nursing Practice*, Robert Wicks specifically addresses the unhealthy culture of healthcare. He defines secondary stress as the pressure that results from reaching out to others in need (e.g., caring for sick patients), which is a constant and continuous reality in medicine, nursing, and allied health. Wicks breaks secondary stress into three components:

- Chronic secondary stress, also known as "burnout"

- Acute secondary stress, also known as vicarious post-traumatic stress disorder (PTSD)
- Other unhealthy aspects of the job unique to the medical healthcare culture

There are multiple manifestations and causes of burnout, but there is one common denominator: "a lack that produces frustration" (Wicks 2005). For nurses, this lack is felt most acutely in the difference between the care nurses believe they should deliver and the care they actually can deliver. Frustrations abound as nurses struggle to obtain the supplies and resources they need to do their jobs.

Other examples of deficiencies surrounding burnout can be the lack of
- breaks
- sufficient staffing
- professional and personal recognition
- education
- coping mechanisms
- staff harmony (Wicks 2005)

In the first phase of burnout, individuals begin to experience emotional exhaustion. Their sense of satisfaction decreases, and they feel drained of energy. These signs and symptoms are "brief in duration and occur only occasionally." In the second phase, nurses develop negative ideas about their patients, coworkers, and themselves. When symptoms become more stable, last longer, and are tougher to get rid of, burnout has progressed to Stage II. By the time a caregiver has reached Stage III, symptoms are chronic and a physical illness has developed (Wicks 2005).

As I read through the definition and causes of burnout, I couldn't help but wonder: *Is horizontal hostility actually a synonym for Stage II burnout?* The major signs and symptoms are familiar—disillusionment, pervasive feelings of frustration or apathy, and intermittent periods of a week or more of feeling irritated, depressed, and stressed. These are the symptoms I observe among my own staff.

Personality style

What personality types are drawn to nursing? In a 1990 study of self-attitudes and behavioral characteristics of Type A and B personalities in female RNs, researchers found that 82% of nurses classified themselves as having a Type A personality (Thomas and Jozwiak 1990). The Type A personality is characterized by hard-driving behavior patterns. Individuals with this personality type are typically very driven (often workaholics), somewhat impatient, and aggressive.

In the study, "Type A nurses scored significantly higher than Type Bs on questions about intense job involvement, speed/impatience, and competitiveness." The researchers also found that "Type A nurses are bringing some attitudes and behaviors with them to the workplace that could kindle angry emotions" and contribute to interpersonal relationship conflict (Thomas and Jozwiak 1990).

"In summary, the Type A RNs appeared to be engaged in competition with time and themselves, as well as competition with other people" (Thomas and Jozwiak 1990). These attitudes come from their belief systems. What are some of the common beliefs of nurses today?

Belief and expectations
Belief systems

In examining our beliefs and expectations, we delve deeper into the causes of frustration in the workplace.

The following are some beliefs that nurses hold:

- *I must have approval from others.*
- *I must be perfect and consider myself inadequate if I make a mistake.*
- *People should be blamed and punished when they do wrong.*
- *It is a catastrophe when things are not as you would like them to be.*
- *Unhappiness is caused by external circumstances beyond your control.*
- *You should worry over possible negative events constantly.*
- *The influence of past events can never be changed or removed.*
- *For every problem, there is a perfect solution that must be found (Thomas 2004).*
- *Compliments are self-aggrandizing.*
- *A good nurse should be able to function on her or his own, without any help.*
- *There is nothing I can do about the situation—that's just the way it is around here.*

What does anger have to do with beliefs? Significant correlations have been found between anger arousal and many irrational beliefs (Thomas 2004). That is, when beliefs don't match reality, we often get angry. When emotions are displaced, misunderstood, and not acknowledged, this anger, as well as a cascade of other conflicting emotions, escalate into horizontal hostility. The following scenarios illustrate the problems that can arise when our beliefs contradict one another and the reality that surrounds us.

Perfectionism: "A good nurse never makes a mistake."
Justice: "Nurses should be punished for mistakes."

It is 2:50, and Martha is in my office just ten minutes before the start of her shift, complaining. Martha tells me that I need to get rid of a new nurse who "does not know what she is doing." She makes no qualms about her intentions—Martha believes that it is her responsibility to oust this new employee in order to uphold the standard of care on the unit.

Ironically, I have a quality variance report on my desk about Martha, who forgot to give coumadin to one patient last night and forgot to chart it for another. This fact does not faze her. She sees absolutely no connection between the other nurse and the fact that she herself is human and has made a mistake as well. Her response to the drug error is, "Oh." Martha continues complaining vehemently about the other nurse. Her belief that nurses must be perfect, and her inability to see her own faults, is unwavering.

Suffering: "A good nurse doesn't mind suffering."
Self-reliance: "A good nurse will never need help."

Alice is in my office for her performance review. I am really struggling with this one. She is an excellent clinical nurse—the best on the floor. But her negativity is toxic, and staff are weary of her constant complaints. "She brings everyone down," they lament.

During the review, I praise her clinical abilities and then pause. Alice is stoic. I can see the wall.

"One more thing, Alice. As you know, I have asked your peers for feedback, and they are very worried." I re-frame her peers' complaints. Half of the wall crumbles.

"You seem so unhappy," I say. "Is there a problem?" Tears flood away the rest of the wall.

Out comes Alice's belief system. That a nurse should be self-sufficient at all times. That asking for help is a sign of weakness. That suffering is next to sainthood. That she should be able to handle everything herself, all the time. "I thought that's what a good nurse was," she says.

Our beliefs are formed from our values. *But these are not our values.* They are the values the dominant group has forced upon our nursing culture: perfectionism, independence, judgment, low self-esteem, and helplessness. **Daily experiences reinforce our belief systems.** Clearly there is an opportunity for nursing leaders not only to bring irrational belief systems to light but also to instill a new set of beliefs based on a new paradigm of an empowered nurse.

Unmet expectations

Years ago, I read a study in *Psychology Today*. The cover page had caught my eye. "What is the most depressing place to live in America?" I thought for sure that the answer would be a very poor part of the country. I was wrong.

Researchers found that the Philadelphia tri-state region was populated by the most depressed people at that time. The reason was because, as young adults, this population expected to have a different lifestyle than their parents—they expected to exceed their parents' lifestyle. But their expectations were dashed as reality—i.e., the high cost of living and a slowing economy—set in. This huge gap between what they expected and what actually happened caused the highest degree of depression.

Coming out of nursing school, our expectations of a nurse's job often present a stark contrast to the reality of nursing. As in the story above, it's not the "worst case scenario" that produces the greatest depression—it's the large gap between expectation and reality. Kramer (1974) found that new graduates experience a "reality shock" that can manifest as hopelessness and dissatisfaction and that these feelings are often a prelude to conflict.

Inadequate communication and conflict management skills
Fear of confrontation and conflict

Anne opens the door to my office. "The patient in 42 says she has not had a bath in two days."

"Well, who had the patient?" I ask.

"Dana."

"Is Dana working today?"

"Yes," she says flatly.

"Well, why don't you ask her about it?"

Now Anne's forehead is all scrunched up. She is not happy. She had already made up her mind (without realizing it) that Dana must have done a poor job. I can hear the judgment in her voice. "What am I supposed to say?" she asks.

"The same thing you just said to me. You say, 'Dana, can I talk to you for a minute? I just came out of 42 and the patient says she has not had a bath in two days.' "

Anne lets out a small groan and leaves reluctantly, as if going for a root canal.

Last year, we had our first charge nurse retreat. It was wonderful. Never before had we been able to simply enjoy each other's presence. On the unit, every conversation seemed to be about staffing shortages or solving patient problems. The retreat, however, gave us the time we so desperately needed to value and appreciate one another.

On this retreat, one of the most amazing eye openers for me, as well as for the charge nurses, was the "leadership cards." In this exercise, nurses selected 20 cards (from a pile of 60) that listed the leadership skills they felt they needed to improve most. The nurses were then asked to pick from this stack of 20 the top three cards they believed would make the biggest difference in their role as charge nurse. Even though all the nurses worked individually for this exercise, *all 11 charge nurses* picked the same card: "Dealing with conflict." Later that day, we did an exercise and went around the room asking, "What drains you? What are circumstances that rob you of your power?"

"I try to hold staff accountable, but some respond so aggressively—they get so angry that it is difficult for me to even approach them . . . so I don't."

"When I see the nursing assistants sitting down and the nurses running around totally overwhelmed, it makes me angry—can't they see? I feel like a nagging mother hounding children all the time. And that doesn't feel good."

"The last time I told an employee that there were way too many personal phone calls at the desk, she punished me! She made my life miserable for weeks by being cold and indifferent."

"Me. I drain me. I put such incredible pressures and unrealistic expectations on myself."

There was a unanimous consensus. Everyone felt that his or her confrontation skills were inadequate. Even the thought of conflict made them cringe, and they had no idea what to say or how to say it. Charge nurses did not have the skills to hold staff accountable. Cohesiveness increased dramatically among the nurses as they identified this common denominator and realized that dealing with conflict was an attainable skill.

Extrinsic factors

"There has been a revolution in medicine concerning how we think about the diseases that now afflict us. It involves recognizing the interactions between the body and the mind, the ways in which emotions and personality can have a tremendous impact on the functioning and health of virtually every cell in the body. It's about the role of stress . . ."
—*Robert Sapolsky,* Why Zebras Don't Get Ulcers

Extrinsic:
- Violent workplace—verbal abuse from patients, families, and physicians
- Poor nurse-physician relationships
- Task and time imperatives—work complexity
- Demands for efficiency/productivity
- Culture

A violent workplace

The United States Department of Justice recorded 429,100 violent crimes against nurses on duty from 1993–1999. "Nurses experienced workplace crime at a rate

72% higher than medical technicians and at twice the rate of other healthcare workers" (Thomas 2004). A study published in the *Journal of Emergency Nursing* in 2002 found that 88% of hospital nurses reported verbal assault and 74% reported being physically assaulted while at work by patients, family members, or visitors in the past year (May and Grubbs 2002).

Why are family members and visitors so angry? The most common reasons for assault included enforcement of hospital policies (58.1%), anger related to the patient's condition (57%), long wait times (47.7%), and anger related in general to the healthcare system (46.5%) (May and Grubbs 2002). Nurses have no control over any of the above issues, but they take the brunt of the anger for them from patients, family, visitors, and, perhaps worst of all, physicians.

Poor nurse-physician relationships

Poor physician-nurse relationships affect morale, patient safety, job satisfaction, and retention (Larson 1999; Rosenstein 2002; Baggs et al. 1999). A 1997 survey published in the *Journal of Professional Nursing* showed that 90% of nurses had witnessed six to 12 unpleasant incidents between physicians and nurses within one year (Manderino and Berkey 1997).

It is no surprise that the most common feeling a nurse experiences after an incident of verbal abuse is anger (Araujo and Sofield 1999). **The term "submissive-aggressive syndrome" is often used to describe the fact that nurses who feel robbed of their power (submissiveness) often react by overpowering others (aggressiveness).** There is no healthy outlet for this anger, so it is seldom expressed except through horizontal hostility. But this form of expression creates a new problem and fails to handle the primary emotion: hurt (Bartholomew 2004).

Task and time imperatives

"I said to the nurse, 'Mrs. Rather needs a bedpan.' But she had no idea who Mrs. Rather was, even though the shift was almost over. The nurse looked at her notes and then finally said, 'Oh, 942.' "

An overload of tasks and time imperatives results in a depersonalization of care. "A nurse's work shift is not finished until all assigned tasks are completed. The nurse who fails to complete his/her tasks at the end of a shift is *persona non grata* (an unwelcome person) to oncoming shift-worker colleagues" (Farrell 2001).

Time and task imperatives are so strong that nurses themselves get trapped in them (Farrell 2001). The focus becomes "what" has to be done in "what" amount of time, and the "who" loses value as tasks accumulate. "So powerful is the notion of task/time imperatives in the nurses' psyche that patients are sometimes seen as tasks, not people" (Farrell 2001). Because of this, we start seeing each other as obstacles instead of human beings. Thus, the new nurse is "in the way." And a nurse has so much on her mind that she refuses help offered to her when she really needs it because to give away a task is to give away control of an extremely delicate operation—her shift.

Even managers, whose job is to streamline efficiency, get caught in the cyclone of activity on the floor and therefore cannot see the complexity of work practices clearly. For example, the morning labs on our unit were drawn around 7 a.m. When the physicians came to the floor, their lab results were not ready, so nurses would call physicians in their offices, or interrupt them in the middle of an operation, just to give them a hematocrit value—on every patient. This practice disrupted the physicians and the nurses, so physicians would often keep nurses on the telephone on hold. Because I was either out on the floor helping the staff or in my office buried in paperwork, it took me two years to see the obvious and to develop a solution: draw the labs at 5 a.m. And then there was the issue of the keys to the patient-controlled analgesic machines—three keys for seven nurses. Issues like these are just the tip of the iceberg. We are so caught up in what needs to be done that we never get a chance to step back and reframe the picture.

Work Complexity

Work complexity is characterized by multiple goals, unpredictability, and constant change. Ebright (2003) and her colleagues found eight patterns that contribute to work complexity: disjointed supply sources, missing equipment, repetitive travel, interruptions, waiting for systems of processes, difficulty accessing resources, inconsistent communication in care, and breakdowns in communication. Up to 40% of a nurse's work is not related to direct care (documenting, learning new technologies). Nurses are interrupted mid-task an average of eight times and experience 8.4 work failures per shift while completing tasks that each take only 3.1 minutes (Tucker). Our units and hospitals are not set up to support the nurse, and the result is often frustration.

We have adapted to the additional stressors in healthcare very poorly: We have become experts at "work-arounds." We have lists of back-door phone numbers and can pull any drug we need from the highly computerized Pyxis machine because we have memorized where that particular drug is (after several incidents of not being able to get the drug when we need it). While these tactics save time, they also increase the probability of committing an error. In haste, we do not double-check our work.

It should not be a major struggle to obtain admission orders for a new patient, stat medications, or a wheelchair for discharge. But it is. Although not necessarily a direct cause of aggression, strict adherence to task/time imperatives "provides the backdrop for situating the occurrence of poor staff relationships within a nursing context" (Farrell 2001). The amount of work we must get done within a particular time frame and our lack of control greatly contribute to our psychological stress.

Increased efficiency = Decreased reflective practice

Nursing today is much too often like working in a "M*A*S*H" unit, with the exception that there is never any time to debrief. At the end of their shifts, nurses spend two minutes reporting the clinical signs, symptoms, and plans of care for their patients. They do this for four to eight patients and then walk out the door—with all of their thoughts and emotions still flaring.

This lack of time for reflection and connection does not allow nurses to make sense of their emotions and leads to isolation, as we believe ourselves to be alone in our anger, depression, frustration, etc. We suffer a tremendous loss when we don't make time for reflective practices and don't listen to ourselves and others. Exchanging our stories would strengthen our bonds and unite us, but instead, we go to battle every day for years without the debriefing that would save our mental health. This lack of connection fosters isolation. When we don't see others in the same boat, we think, feel, and become life preservers, just looking after ourselves.

Pat is the charge nurse and, at 7:45 a.m., is already in her manager's office venting. "And Kim is still mad! What else am I supposed to do?"

A few hours later, her manager is rounding and runs into Kim. The manager is direct. "I heard you have a heavy load but that Pat can help you." Kim looks overwhelmed, so the manager asks if there is anything she can do.

"Yes," she replies, "you can listen to me."

As Kim's story unfolds, the manager learns that Kim's nursing assistant did not show up until 8:15 a.m. and that no one had mentioned to her that she was going to be late. Kim explains that she then asked a preceptee to hang the blood, but the preceptor said her preceptee already had enough experience, etc., etc.

"I'm sorry," the manager replies. "Let's meet with Pat after the shift."

But Pat does not want to meet. She is very tired and near tears, and all she wants to do is go home. Eleven surgeries have rolled back on the floor, and she is worried about her son, who is away at college. She is frustrated because she cannot make things better. It just seems like it never ends, and the support she offers to others is worthless. Kim, however, insists, and the two come into the manager's office.

Kim is the first to start. She tells Pat how much she respects her and that she thinks the world of her and her leadership skills, but that she is really mad that no one told her that Jennifer, her nursing assistant, would be so late. As it turns out, Kim is angry with Pat because of this, but instead of telling her, she complained about another assignment.

Pat had no idea about Kim's true compliant. She heard the secretary say, "Jennifer will be late," but thought she meant Jennifer the educator, not Jennifer Kim's nursing assistant. In turn, Pat became angry because she had worked so hard to make a fair report and provide resources, yet was treated so harshly.

The conversation only touches the surface. Strong feelings of betrayal lie underneath.

The next layer reveals that Kim was angry about attending a preceptor workshop that Pat had signed her up for that same day. Out comes another story—the real reason *behind all the conflict of the day. Angrily, Kim explains to Pat, "It was passive-aggressive of you to sign me up for that preceptor class because you thought I was awful."*

As the manager asks what she means, more gossip rises to the surface. Kim had heard a rumor that she was too hard on the new preceptees. So if that was true, why were we sending her to a preceptor workshop—was it some kind of joke? So much pain . . .

In this debriefing, both nurses had the opportunity to express themselves, and the end result was a great deal of understanding and empathy for one another. It was clear that Kim felt devalued and unrecognized for her precepting on the floor. And she was hurt. The rumblings of the day signaled a much larger emotional issue. Everyone on the floor was aware of the drama and its impact on the atmosphere of the unit, but emotions were so strong and everyone was so busy that the issue was avoided. Had this conversation never happened, an undercurrent of anger would have permeated the floor for weeks or even months. The destructive effect on morale and teamwork would have been horrendous.

Culture

"Why would I want to go to college [and become a nurse] so that someone else can tell me what to do all the time?"

—A nurse's daughter

Our profession was designed to mimic the military model—even our terminology reflects it: surgeon general, charge nurse, post op *orders*. In phenomenological interviews, military metaphors permeate the conversations. Nurses described themselves as "under assault" in a hostile environment (Smith et al. 1996). I can recall a nurse on our floor looking at her schedule and upon realizing that she would be on duty for all three days of our JCAHO visit said, "I want combat pay"—only half joking.

In line with this model is nurses' lack of autonomy to make independent decisions. Yet autonomy (control over practice) has been shown to be the most important factor in job satisfaction for nurses (Dunn 2003). Physicians give inconsistent responses to nurses who demonstrate autonomy. Depending on the severity of the situation or the time of day, nurses are either applauded or condemned for their independent problem-solving actions; the same physician who applauds a nurse for not calling at midnight will turn around and chastise her for exercising independent thinking during the day. This inconsistency discourages nurses from acting autonomously and leads to hyper-vigilance (Gordon 2005).

Every profession has a unique culture. The military model is not attractive to new nurses because it squashes autonomy, which is key to job and staff satisfaction.

In addition, the nursing culture has historically lacked a constructive way to give feedback. Nurses who have worked with each other for 20 years have never been asked to give feedback about their peers, charge nurses, or managers. Because we are human beings, if there is no way to give constructive feedback we often turn to off-hand comments as the only way to express our opinion. Professionals, however, solicit the input of their peers in order to obtain as much information as possible so that they can more accurately perceive themselves and identify areas for improvement. The very act of asking for this information debunks the myth that we are perfect.

Summary

Intrinsic and extrinsic factors play major roles in perpetuating horizontal hostility. Horizontal hostility may have its roots in oppression, but there are clearly other forces that fan the flames: a violent workplace, disenfranchising work practices, emotional angst, verbal abuse from physicians, Type A personality traits, unrealistic beliefs, unmet expectations, and poor confrontation skills.

Although horizontal hostility occurs in all service-oriented industries, it is especially virulent in healthcare. After examining the intrinsic and extrinsic factors that add momentum to normalized behaviors, our focus now turns to a broader context—horizontal hostility in the context of the organizational structure, our profession, and our world.

Bibliography

Aiken, L., et al. 2002. Hospital Nurse Staffing and Patient Mortality, Nurse Burnout, and Job Dissatisfaction. *Journal of the American Medical Association* 288: 1987–1993.

Araujo, S., and L. Sofield. 1999. Verbal abuse. *http://home.comcast.net/~laura 08723/survey.htm.*

Baggs, J. et al. 1999. Association between nurse-physician collaboration and patient outcomes in three intensive care units. *Critical Care Medicine* 27(9): 1998–1999.

Bartholomew, K. 2004. *Speak Your Truth: Proven strategies for effective nurse-physician communication.* Marblehead, MA: HCPro, Inc.

Dunn, H. 2003. Horizontal violence among nurses in the operating room. *AORN Journal* 78(6).

Ebright, P. et al. 2003. Understanding the complexity of registered nurse work in acute care settings. *Journal of Nursing Administration,* Vol. 33. No. 12.

Erickson, R., Grove, W. 2007. Why emotions matter: age, agitation, and burn-out among registered nurses. *The Online Journal of Issues in Nursing.* Available at *www.nursingworld.org/MainMenuCategories/ANAMarketplace/ANAPeriodicals/OJIN/TableofContents/Volume62001/Number1January2001/WhyEmotionsMatterAgeAgitation andBurnoutAmongRegisteredNurses.aspx.*

Farrell, G. 2001. From tall poppies to squashed weeds: Why don't nurses pull together more? *Journal of Advanced Nursing* 35(1): 26–33.

Gordon, S. 2005. *Nursing Against the Odds: How Health Care Cost Cutting, Media Stereotypes, and Medical Hubris Undermine Nurses and Patient Care (The Culture and Politics of Health Care Work).* Ithaca, NY: ILR Press.

Kramer, M. 1974. *Reality Shock: Why nurses leave nursing* (1 ed.). St. Louis, MO: The C.V. Mosby Company.

Larson, E. 1999. The impact of physician-nurse interaction on patient care. *Holistic Nursing Practice* 13(2): 38–47.

Manderino, M., and N. Berkey. 1997. Verbal abuse of staff nurses by physicians. *Journal of Professional Nursing* 13(1): 48–55.

May, D., and L. Grubbs. 2002. The extent, nature, and precipitating factors of nurse assault among three groups of registered nurses in a regional medical center. *Journal of Emergency Nursing* 28(3): 191.

Rosenstein, A. 2002. Nurse-physician relationships: impact on nurse satisfaction and retention. *Advanced Journal of Nursing* 102(6): 26–34.

Sapolsky, R. 1998. *Why Zebras Don't Get Ulcers: An updated guide to stress, stress-related diseases and coping.* New York: Freeman & Company.

Smith, M., P. Droppleman, and S. Thomas. 1996. Under assault: The experience of work-related anger in female registered nurses. *Nursing Forum* 31(1): 22–33.

Thomas, S. 2004. *Transforming Nurses' Stress and Anger: Steps toward healing.* New York: Springer Publishing Company.

Thomas, S., and J. Jozwiak. 1990. Self attitudes and behavioral characteristics of Type A and B female registered nurses. *Health Care for Women International* 11: 477–489.

Tucker, A.L., Spear S.J. 2006. Operational failures and interruptions in hospital nursing. *Health Services Research*. June; 41:643-62.

Wicks, R. 2005. *Overcoming Secondary Stress in Medical and Nursing Practice.* United Kingdom: Oxford University Press.

Enlarging the landscape

Context is critical

All five children are yelling, and the sound just seems more amplified by the tin walls of our single-wide trailer. Everyone is trying to stake out their own territory in our new space and, clearly, it's not working.

"Stop!" I scream. "Sit down—now!"

I can tell from their anxious faces that they expect admonishment (and, indeed, that is exactly what I had planned). But suddenly a story comes to mind, and I decide to trust it.

"Once upon a time, there was a researcher who loved mice. Every day he happily added another mouse to his cage. Suddenly, when the cage became jammed with a certain number of mice, the researcher was shocked to discover that the mice actually started killing each other."

The trailer is quiet. After a long pause, Katie, age 7, asks, "What does that mean?"

"It means," I say calmly, "go outside and play."

To view horizontal hostility solely in the context of an individual nurse on a nursing unit is limiting and one-dimensional. In order to recognize all the factors that contribute to hostility, we need to expand our focus and examine hostility in three separate yet interwoven contexts: the organizational context, the professional context, and the context of our world. Only by stepping back and enlarging the landscape can leaders develop the wisdom and compassion they need to create a culture of respect.

Organizational context

Hostility is a natural outcome of working in a hierarchical system where there is little control and scarce resources—the United States healthcare system. By its very nature, the structure of the healthcare system supports oppression. Hierarchy squashes autonomy, diminishes pride and identity, and silences voice.

Oppression is the product of a system that does not work. *Everyone* who works in a hospital feels its effects, and, ultimately, so does the patient. The current workload demands that nurses focus on what is directly in front of them, but what can we learn if we zoom out from the unit where a staff nurse is currently belittling her coworker? **What does horizontal hostility look like in the context of a hospital?**

As CEO of a large tertiary hospital, Robert is preparing for his quarterly meeting with the Board of Directors. Unconsciously, he takes a deep breath and stares at the neatly stacked reports piled on his desk. As hospital margins shrink, the cost of doing business rises sharply every year. Medicare reimbursement rates are down to 42 cents on the dollar, the hospital insurance policy deductible has increased 100 fold (from last year's deductible of 1,000 to 100,000), the union is bargaining for higher wages and a better insurance package, and the number of uninsured cases has increased. Several years ago, Robert eliminated the Chief Nursing Officer and other administrative positions due to advice he had read on hospital restructuring and reorganization in the late 1990s. To make matters worse, patients are now asking for outcomes and satisfaction measurements, and Robert must keep these scores high in order to stay competitive. Frustrated and challenged from all directions, his eyes rivet on the only pile he can control. Robert cuts a half-million dollars from nursing and support services, just as he did last year.

Alex sits at his desk scouring the fourth quarter service excellence reports. As Vice President of Quality, he is responsible for creating a culture of excellence and does not understand why the numbers haven't changed in almost two years. Even the employee and physician satisfaction scores have not improved despite a massive campaign to uphold new behavioral standards of customer service. The hospital has invested heavily in consultants to get this project off the ground. Each manager must send thank you notes, round with staff, post strategic action plans, and report back—but the numbers just aren't moving. He shoots an urgent e-mail to his director, requesting a meeting.

Eleanor is in charge of the service excellence and service recovery program. She is responsible for compiling all the system-wide reports and presenting them to hospital employees and senior leadership. She has poured a lot of time and energy into making the service excellence program succeed by developing campaigns and presenting at meetings. Two of her employees have been out sick on FMLA and, unbeknownst to her, the one remaining employee, Carol, is ready to quit at any minute. Feeling unheard and unsupported, Carol heads to her meeting with Jane, her manager, to resolve a patient complaint—and do some complaining herself.

Jane slams the file cabinet door shut in frustration. For eight years, she has been writing reports, sending e-mails, and reporting to her boss that she needs more resources to operate the floor, more personnel, and an education space for her elective surgery patients. She has tried to see all 70 patients every week as the service excellence commitments dictate, but that has meant coming in on weekends. Yesterday, she spent almost an hour dealing with an angry patient who did not understand why he didn't routinely receive pain mediations every three hours. Another patient's anxiety level was so high that he had a panic attack as soon he hit the floor from surgery. If only they knew what to expect, she wouldn't be spending all her time explaining procedures and protocols to patients who were half-drugged on pain meds anyway! Just then, one of Jane's nurses opens the door with a question on the service excellence report.

"Excuse me," the nurse says, "How many discharge phone calls did we make this month?"

Jane is overwhelmed. She sighs and replies, "Pick a number." The floor is two nurses short for evening shift, and she has already called several nurses, but no one wants to work. Maybe Kim can double?

Kim is clearly irritated by the time report ends. "I have two amputees and my nursing assistant was late," she complains to the charge nurse.

"Don't worry. I'll help you, and Stephanie's preceptee can help too," the charge nurse replies.

But things just get worse. When Kim asks Stephanie if her preceptee can hang a unit of blood, Stephanie retorts, "She already knows how to do that." Kim is irritated. "Some help," she mutters.

As Kim approaches the main nursing station, she sees that the charge nurse is now making discharge phone calls and is unable to help. Irritated, she turns and barks an order at the nursing assistant who had shown up late.

"Hurry up, the cabulance is coming at 11 and Mr. Walker must be ready!"

The cabulance driver arrives on the floor to pick up Mr. Walker, only to find him in a dirty gown. It's 11:00 a.m., and he has not yet had breakfast. In the commotion that follows as staff race to make last-minute preparations, no one notices that Mr. Walker puts a call in to his friend—on the Board of Directors.

Oppression results as the pressures of working in an inefficient and costly system are passed down from one level to another. Oppression is felt in every tier, but its effects are frequently not acknowledged because of intense work demands. In large organizations, this is often the point of disconnect, as staff are so consumed by their individual task and time imperatives that they fail to see the big picture or hear the needs of the subordinate group. It's a one-way conversation: down.

How the organizational structure enables oppression

"The problem is that hospital restructuring has fundamentally changed organizational arrangements that shape nurses' daily work lives and what it means to be a nurse."

—Dana Beth Weinberg, Code Green

Healthcare is a business because its very existence depends on its ability to be financially viable. Add to the typical characteristics inherent in businesses a set of governmental controls, and the result is rules, regulations, and a rigid system of bureaucratic hierarchy. As we descend the ladder of hierarchy, the pressure (or oppression) increases in both frequency and intensity for two reasons. First, the lower down you go on the food chain, the thicker the veil of oppression. Nurses, who are situated at the bottom of the ladder, are so absorbed in the tasks directly in front of them that they do not have time for reflective practice, which would allow them to deal with their emotional state. We can't fight what we can't see. A behavior not named is an invisible dragon.

The second reason that nursing feels such intense oppression is because nurses are feeling the *total weight* of all the pressures from above. Situated at the bottom of the hierarchical ladder, nursing absorbs the cumulative pressures of the organization. The stresses that Robert feels are passed down to Alex, who has his own set of pressures from previous cutbacks and who passes all that down to Eleanor, and so forth. And because nursing is multidisciplinary, it feels pressure from all directions. For example, having no discharge social worker on Saturdays means the nurse must stop and arrange the cabulance; having no nutrition services after 9 p.m. forces the nurse to fix the snacks, etc. Nurses constantly absorb others' work without additional resources and fail to evaluate the effect this has on nursing practice.

Another characteristic of horizontal hostility is that it is insidious—it spreads harmfully in a subtle manner. To say that the veil of oppression keeps us hidden is extremely accurate: Not only are nurses prevented from seeing clearly out through the veil, but the dominant group cannot see in either.

Administration cannot respond to the needs of a group characterized by silence and invisibility. Nurses immersed in a drama often take negative comments personally and spend their energy licking their own wounds. Alternatively, nurses ignore their wounds because they are too busy. In addition to the general lack of voice, those who do speak are often labeled as not being "team players" in the nursing culture and are left feeling unheard and invalidated.

A conflict of interests

The fact that healthcare is a business produces a conflict of interests. Nurses' greatest desire is to provide high quality care, but although quality is also a goal of the institution, it is not the institution's *primary* goal. Rather, a hospital's primary goal is to stay financially viable. This conflict of primary interests produces a profound power struggle.

The pressures passed down by the organization are essentially the result of a struggle for a limited amount of power. In her book, *Code Green: Money-driven Hospitals and the Dismantling of Nursing*, Dana Beth Weinberg discusses power as related to hospital mergers and points out that power is *situational*. We can view this power in two ways: as a finite (limited) amount or an expanding amount (Katz and Kahn 1978). Whether power is finite or expanding depends on whether there is commonality or a conflict of interests; when there is a difference in primary objectives (i.e., a conflict of interests), power is perceived as finite (Weinberg 2003). Because we know that a conflict of interests does exist between healthcare and nursing, we can conclude that only a limited amount of power lies between these two groups. This results in a struggle for power, which administration undeniably wins, leaving nurses feeling powerless.

"What bothers me the most is that I come with the room charge—like a bed or a water pitcher . . . I am insulted because there is nothing that differentiates me from 'things.' "

Because healthcare is a business, nurses are viewed as an interchangeable commodity. "If those who work within the acute healthcare bureaucracy are identified as a commodity rather than a valued asset, there can be a sense of helplessness, lack of autonomy, and perception of no respect arising from a profound feeling of powerlessness" (Sumner and Townsend-Rocchiccioli 2003).

Professional context

Horizontal hostility is not only inherent in the organizational structure but also stems from conflict within our profession. The most obvious of these conflicts is the profession's lack of consensus concerning the entry-level requirement for nursing—ADN or BSN.

Less obvious, however, is the conflict in the very nature of our work. In his book, *Beyond Caring: Hospitals, Nurses and the Social Organization of Ethics,* Daniel Chambliss identifies three core features of nurses' work, which he labels "missions." The nurse is expected, and typically expects herself, to simultaneously be a

1. caring individual
2. professional
3. relatively subordinate member of the organization

But there is a problem. "The directives conflict: be caring and yet professional; be subordinate and yet responsible, be diffusely accountable for a patient's well-being and yet oriented to the hospital as an economic employer" (Chambliss 1996).

Code Green gives an important and detailed account of how hospital cost-cutting and downsizing as a response to managed care in the late 1990s magnified this conflict. "In particular, hospital restructuring devalued the caring aspects of nurses' role, strained their ability to act as professionals, and emphasized their subordination to institutions that find it necessary to emphasize margin over mission" (Weinberg 2003).

Our fundamental desire to be caring and professional, yet also subordinate, causes a great deal of inner turmoil on a daily basis. Nurses function in a subordinate position with unrealistic institutional expectations. We spend a lot of wasted energy trying to get the resources we need to do our job. We are expected to continuously provide a certain standard of care—indeed "ordered to care in a society that refuses to value caring" (Reverby 1987).

Caring is one of the fundamental tenets of nursing. By caring, we create and hold a space so that our patients can heal. It is emotional work. When our hearts are wounded, the care we deliver is far from optimal. If we are upset, we can't think straight. No nurse, especially those at the first line of defense—the bedside—can afford for this to happen. **The mental and emotional state of nurses is a critical human factor.** There is an obvious and direct link between our emotions and our mental clarity—and our mental clarity and patient safety.

Don Berwick, MD, MPP, cofounder of the Institute for Healthcare Improvement (IHI) in Boston, is well known for saying, "Every system is perfectly designed to produce the results it consistently achieves." This statement was first applied in the automobile industry to illustrate that car quality was a direct result of the factory process. We know the results in healthcare:

- 48,000–98,000 patients die every year from medical errors.
- Nurses are dissatisfied and leaving while
  - -we face the worst nursing shortage in history, while
  - -we deal with having an inadequate number of faculty.

In the Aiken study, which examined the link between nurse-to-patient ratio and patient deaths, as well as factors related to RN retention, Aiken and her colleagues found that "higher emotional exhaustion and greater job dissatisfaction were significantly associated with patient-to-nurse ratios." The study linked data from 10,184 staff nurses to 232,342 general, orthopedic, and vascular patients in 1999. For each additional patient over four in a nurse's workload, the risk of death increased by 7% for surgical patients. If the nurse-to-patient ratio was 1:8, patients had a 31% greater risk of dying. "On a national scale, staffing differences of this magnitude may result in as many as 20,000 unnecessary deaths each year" (Aiken et al. 2002). The study also left no doubt that there is a link between staffing levels, burnout, and job satisfaction.

No one will debate that the system is not working. Yet despite these well-known facts, the public is not up in arms. And although nurses constitute a significant enough percentage of the population to take a strong stand themselves, nurses have not united to address the problem. **Horizontal hostility is a critical impediment to solidarity.** It is the antithesis of teamwork. If nurses are not speaking out in one unified voice to change the system, then what are nurses saying? Until we begin to listen and make our voices heard, it will be impossible to unite to address the bigger issues.

In her book, *Transforming Nurses' Stress and Anger: Steps Toward Healing*, Sandra Thomas summarizes the themes that emerged from years of gathering nurses' stories about their stress and anger:

- *"I feel overloaded and overwhelmed."*
- *"I am not treated with respect."*
- *"I am blamed and scapegoated."*
- *"I feel powerless."*
- *"I am not being heard."*
- *"I feel morally sick."*
- *"I am not getting any support." (Thomas 2004)*

The powerlessness and helplessness expressed in these statements is overwhelming. But these are not the only stressors nurses feel. If we expand our focus to include the daily challenges of living in the present day in the United States, it is easy to see why "everyday nursing" can feel like an emotional percolator.

In the context of our world

I have always considered myself the queen of multitasking—the divine diva of efficiency. So last summer, I had carefully calculated that I had just enough time before my 2:00 p.m. meeting to take my son to the doctor. He had injured his shoulder in the spring, and months later it was still hurting. As I got into the car at the parking garage, I saw the yellow sticky I had carefully placed on the dashboard earlier that day that read, "Don't forget the x-rays." No problem, I thought. Last night I had done a visual check and they were behind the bookcase.

Everything was running smoothly until the moment the doctor held up the x-rays to the light. At first he scrunched up his face. Then, with a straight face, he turned to me and said, "Mrs. Bartholomew, I have some bad news. Your son is a small dog."

In my haste and efficiency, I had grabbed the dog's x-rays instead of my son's.

No one comes to work and leaves all of their problems at home. We can't swipe in our badges and simultaneously wipe out our minds, deleting all the things we worry about outside of work. Nurses bring their problems with them to the workplace.

"The year 2000 marked the first time that less than a quarter (23.5%) of American households were made up of a married man and woman and one or more children—a drop from 45% in 1960. The number is expected to fall to 20% by 2010" (Sado and Bayer 2001). These numbers mean that nurses are often single parents who carry additional responsibilities that add additional stressors to everyday life. Phone calls interrupt a nurse's daily routine as she tries to figure out who can pick Johnny up from school and then who will take care of him until she gets home.

Additionally, for the first time in history, our children are sicker than their parents (McDonough 2002). The largest growing segment of the population for prescription drugs is children under the age of 19—despite the fact that the 65+ generation has grown by 10% (Putnam 2000). Some of the major problems these drugs are addressing in young people are hyperactivity, depression, high blood pressure, and diabetes.

"When I hurt myself at work, to tell you the truth, it was a relief. I had to stay home for three weeks. I got to stop. I got to remember what 'stop' was."

Furthermore, membership in both professional and recreational groups has decreased significantly in the last fifty years (Putnam 2000). We are simply too busy for it. As a result, our social support group is faltering, and we are becoming more isolated. Social skills normally practiced in group settings are declining. The pressures of our life mount with the realization that we are "on our own."

One of the most important indicators of intent to stay is a sense of belonging. How important is belonging? "Joining any group at all cuts in half your chances of dying" (Putnam 2000). But you can't belong to a group if no one knows you, if no one ever has any downtime, or if the pace of work is so intense you can't get a break or eat lunch. Yet the majority of us spend more time with our coworkers in any given week than we do with our families.

"If I do get a break, I use that time to make appointments for car repairs or doctor visits for the kids. When I ride the ferry to work, I use that time to pay my bills."

In 1965, economists predicted that in the year 2000, Americans would have more than 600 *billion* hours of additional leisure time due to all of the time-saving inventions of that period. How are we spending our time? Instead of vacationing, we now work 60+ hours a week. According to the Stanford Institute for the Quantitative Study of Society, Americans spend an average of three hours a day on the Internet. Our "speed dialing, speed dating, fast track, express line, quickie mart" life is taking its toll.

Nurses feel the stressors of their organization, their profession, and their world—and don't always deal with them in a healthy manner. The American Nurses Association (ANA) estimates that 6%–8% of nurses use alcohol or other drugs to the extent that they impair their professional performance.

The average age of a nurse (48 years) has risen sharply over the past few years, primarily due to the nursing shortage. Most of these nurses have a 20+ year career, and the physical and mental wear and tear on their bodies has had a cumulative effect. Nurses are experiencing injuries that they are not reporting to their hospitals due to labor-intensive paperwork and the inability find a physician who accepts Labor and Industry compensation. Administration cannot address a problem it does not know exists.

Summary

Viewing hostility in the context of the organization, our profession, and our world gives us some additional clues about why horizontal hostility occurs. In our current healthcare system, nurses suffer from a profound sense of powerlessness, a lack of autonomy, decreased job satisfaction and morale, and a weak identity. These characteristics are all associated with oppressed groups.

From applying the oppression theory, we know that
- in-fighting is a known attribute of any oppressed group
- attributes originally valued by the subordinate group are devalued
- this devaluation manifests itself in low self-esteem

From studying animals, we know that

- primates are known for displacing aggression
- three factors increase psychological stress
  - -the lack of an outlet for frustration
  - -the lack of social support systems
  - -unpredictability

From an organizational and professional context, we know horizontal hostility emerges due to

- a lack of voice or representation in the organization's hierarchical structure
- a conflict of primary interests with the dominant group
- a constant power struggle for finite resources
- increasing pressure on hospitals to survive financially (which is heavily felt on the bottom tier—nursing)
- a lack of solidarity within our own profession, which prevents mobilization of resources

From the context of the world we live in, we know that

- nurses face mounting pressures in their personal lives
- there has been a significant decrease in social support networks
- staff bring outside pressures to the workplace

Recommended reading

Code Green: Money-Driven Hospitals and the Dismantling of Nursing
  By Dana Beth Weinberg

*Nursing Against the Odds: How Health Care Cost Cutting, Media Stereotypes, and
Medical Hubris Undermine Nurses and Patient Care*
  By Suzanne Gordon

Transforming Nurses' Stress and Anger: Steps Toward Healing
  By Sandra P. Thomas

Bibliography

Aiken, L. et al. 2002. Hospital Nurse Staffing and Patient Mortality, Nurse
Burnout, and Job Dissatisfaction. *Journal of the American Medical Association*
288(16).

Chambliss, D. 1996. *Beyond Caring: Hospitals, Nurses and the Social Organization of
Ethics.* Chicago, IL: University of Chicago Press.

Gordon, S. 2005. *Nursing Against the Odds: How health care cost cutting, media stereotypes, and medical hubris undermine nurses and patient care.* Ithaca, NY: ILR Press.

Katz, D., and R. Kahn. 1978. *The Social Psychology of Organizations.* Second
Edition. New York: Wiley.

McDonough, W. 2002. Institute of Noetic Sciences Conference. Palm Springs, CA.

Putnam, R. 2000. *Bowling Alone: The collapse and revival of American community*. New York: Simon & Schuster.

Reverby, S. 1987. *Ordered to Care: The dilemma of American nursing 1850–1945*. New York: Cambridge University Press.

Sado, S., and A. Bayer. 2001. Executive Summary: The Changing American Family. Population Resource Center.

Sumner, J., and J. Townsend-Rocchiccioli. 2003. Why are nurses leaving nursing? *Nursing Administration Quarterly* 27(2): 164–171.

Thomas, S. 2004. *Transforming Nurses' Stress and Anger: Steps Toward Healing*. New York: Springer Publishing Company.

Weinberg, D. 2003. *Code Green: Money driven hospitals and the dismantling of nursing*. Ithaca, NY: Cornell University Press.

Best practices to eliminate horizontal hostility

Best practices to eliminate horizontal hostility

Introduction

"I remain convinced that a transformation must take place in nursing, a transformation in the hearts and minds of individual nurses that ultimately creates peace and harmony in our relationships with one another. If we do not link arms to face today's formidable challenges, nursing's future could be in jeopardy."

—S. Thomas

The question is: how do we change course? Given the increasing pressures on everyone in nursing, from university professors to student nurses, it seems that our energy can best be spent in a unified, passionate, and immediate response. Understanding the forces that contribute to horizontal hostility (Section I) was the first step. Taking action is the second (Section II).

Just as Section I gave us a conceptual framework for understanding horizontal hostility, Section II provides us with a conceptual framework for the solution. **Our solution lies in the etiology, or study of causation, of the problem.**

Therefore, we must recognize that

- because hierarchy diminishes two-way communication and power, **leveling the playing field will decrease hostility**

- because powerlessness is a result of an unequal, finite amount of power, **empowering nurses and encouraging voice will decrease hostility**

- because silence and closed systems perpetuate horizontal hostility, **creating an environment where staff feel free to communicate (to speak their truth) is critical**

- because horizontal hostility is insidious, **bringing the subject out into the open will decrease its prevalence**

- because decreased self-esteem is a common theme in oppressed groups (and because it maintains the status quo), **any intervention directed at increasing esteem will decrease horizontal hostility**

- because pressure has increased in the workplace and we have adapted to a great deal of unconscious stressors, **stopping to acknowledge these pressures will increase awareness and decrease frustration/hostility**

- because a faster pace of work does not allow us time to see the consequences of our actions, **reflective practice will allow us an opportunity to see how our behaviors affect each other and decrease hostility**

- because a belief system of subordination accompanies oppression, **illuminat-**

**ing these beliefs and creating a new archetype will foster healthy
work attitudes**

- because the lack of a social support network increases aggression, **increasing
social support networks will decrease psychological stress**

The following chapters contain specific examples and interventions for building a
healthy work culture and decreasing horizontal hostility. The common denominator in all of these interventions will be

- leveling the playing field (i.e., decreasing stratification)
- empowering staff by increasing voice or agency
- raising awareness
- increasing self-esteem
- creating an open communication network
- providing opportunities for reflection
- increasing social support networks
- illuminating the problem by bringing the consequences into the open

We can only take action to the extent that we can distance ourselves from the
problem. This distance from the drama, or the emotional issues of our workplace,
gives us a new perspective empowered with solutions. As leaders, we are keenly
aware of the pressures of working in healthcare, but we are extremely engaged
in day-to-day operations. To heal horizontal hostility, we need to step out of
this world . . .

The big picture: An analogy

Actors: our feelings; **acting out** the hostile behavior

Audience: the part of ourselves that **reflects** on our actions

Director: our thinking self; the part of ourselves that **critically analyzes** and has the ability to delete, add lines, or write a new script

Think of a large Opera House.

In the Opera House are many theatres, and in each theatre a play is **NOW SHOWING!**

In Theatre Number One, *Horizontal Hostility* is playing. This drama began decades ago as a one act play called *Join Us if You Can*, featuring new nurses being educated into the hospital setting. Nobody remembers who wrote that script—probably because it was a doctor.

About ten years ago, the play became a full-length feature portraying the intense drama in the relationships among nurses and was renamed *Horizontal Hostility*. You have to be really smart to get a role in this play—and have a very large bladder capacity, because there are no bathroom breaks. If you can find the time to eat something, you won't remember what you ate because you are too busy concentrating on juggling your responsibilities.

All the actors are playing nurses. Some actors have main roles, some play supporting roles, and some you can't distinguish from the scenery. Nurses learn their lines as understudies, so the nonstop acting has been able to run continuously for years. This is primarily because when you have a play going 24 hours a day, you can't stop the momentum. Like a merry-go-round that's always spinning, actors learn how to jump on and off on cue.

There is no audience. After you play a role for 40,000 or so hours like most of the crew, you forget about the audience because the play itself requires so much energy.

In Theatre Number Two, *A Day in the Life of a Manager* is playing. New actresses for this role are just thrown on stage and learn by improvising. Usually, you can get a job here very easily because there is never a waiting list. The action is intense—stand-up tragedy. When the play was popular 20 years ago, some of the managers could take a break and go see *Horizontal Hostility,* but that hasn't happened for a long time.

No one can remember an audience. It's even hard for the managers to remember where they parked their cars because it's usually dark out when they start and dark again when they go home. If you miss your cue (or just admit that you can never find your car), you lose your role. Most people think that's a bad thing.

In Theatre Number Three and Four are the directors and administrators—all very involved in their own dramas, but with a *much bigger orchestra.* There are no props, and the scenery is bleak. They can't miss a beat and the music never stops. It is virtually impossible for anyone to step out of their role or they might miss some critical dialogue in the play, so nobody has left the stage for a long time. They don't break to eat, nor do they show any emotion, which has led some outsiders to wonder if they are even human.

In the last Theatre is the CEO. He's doing a soliloquy—available on DVD.

From the audience, the impact of horizontal hostility is clear. Stepping out of the play and into the audience is the only way we can understand the drama. Only from this perspective can we reflect on our actions. This is how we illuminate the behavior. By doing so, we see that there is indeed a larger setting. We can anticipate the next scene and realize the effect horizontal hostility has on all the characters—pain.

If we can simply step out of the drama long enough to find the director—that part of ourselves that can write a new script—we can end the cycle of hostility.

Everyday,
in every interaction,
we either approve of the old script
or write a new one.

Nurturing our young

"The profession of nursing has an obligation to reduce lateral violence. The population of newly registered nurses is an ideal place to start. They collectively represent the profession of the future."

—Griffin (2004)

It is time to build a new archetype: an ideal of nursing whose belief system empowers nurses and recognizes the unique and critical role they play in our society. A logical place to start is with the new generation of nurses. Our sincere gratitude for choosing nursing must become a hallmark of our mentoring.

Of critical importance in the nursing shortage is the fact that "60% of newly registered nurses leave their first position within six months because of some form of lateral violence perpetrated against them" (Griffin 2004). Researchers in New Zealand found that horizontal hostility is a common experience for first-year nurses and that half of the horizontal hostility new graduates experienced was not reported. In addition, researchers found that these new nurses lacked the skills needed to deal with hostility (McKenna et al. 2003).

"My orientation was spent crying in the bathroom. The strange part was that no one did anything about the behavior. The manager felt that we had a communication problem and that we didn't understand each other—a 'personality conflict.' "

"Everything about [the ICU nurse's] tone was condescending. The message was loud and clear, but unspoken. She was precepting a new nurse, and as soon as she saw me she started putting me down, as if to make it clear that there was a hierarchy even within nursing—that an ICU nurse was much more important than a floor nurse."

Impediments to a healthy new nurse experience

Staff workload

Downsizing in hospitals has forced employees to take on multiple new tasks, often with a decrease in available resources and an increase in job complexity (Keuter et al. 2000). The result is an increased workload. "Experienced nurses who are already working in stressful conditions with continuous staff shortages and poor recognition of service see the student nurse sometimes as an extra hindrance to their already increasing workload" (Davey 2002).

"Due to the 'grid,' when I am precepting a new nurse, I still have the same number of patients that I do every other day. It's ridiculous. If someone just followed me for a day, they would see that I can't give these new nurses the attention they deserve."

Over the years, experienced nurses have picked up new ways of coping with the stress of their workload. I inadvertently discovered one of these "innovative" approaches one day when I met with a student nurse and a preceptor to find out more details about a medication error that had occurred. The student had given the wrong medication to the wrong patient and the instructor had called me, alarmed. As it turned out, the precepting nurse had taught the student her "short cut": She was pulling out pills before they were due on a patient and keeping them in her pocket.

Erroneous assumptions

Every day in nursing brings incremental pressures that were not there the day before: escalating acuity, physically heavier patients, shorter lengths of stay, new technology and treatments, and higher staff ratios. Advances in technology and pharmacology have resulted in an increase in pills and information that challenges even experienced nurses. Therefore, from a clinical standpoint, new resident nurses are not walking into the same scenario as their mentors.

One would think that experienced nurses would welcome new grads in a nursing shortage. Last year, I decided to put a new resident nurse into the hands of one of our younger nurses who had been with us for five years. Her lack of patience and harsh expectations took me by surprise. After speaking to the nurse, I learned her underlying belief system: "If I did it, she can too. If I had to do orientation in 12 weeks, so should she." This could be considered a "hazing" or induction phase, which is also commonly practiced among physicians. In every comment, the nurse was comparing the new resident nurse to herself and to her own experience.

New nurse perceptions

Studies show that the number one clinical teaching behavior that students seek in their instructors is approachability, followed by fairness, openness, honesty, and mutual respect (Viverais-Dresler and Kutschke 2001). Yet as the pace of work on the floor increases, nurses become less approachable than ever—and difficult to connect with because they don't slow down. Time to bond has decreased as nurses skip meals and social interaction dwindles.

Lacking an understanding of the pace of the floor and the intensity of the workload, new nurses believe that they are "in the way," which often leads to feelings of rejection and a lack of the bonding that is so critical to new grads. In addition, the whining and complaining new nurses hear from others causes them to question their choice of nursing as a career.

Creating a healthy environment for student nurses

Consider using the following strategies to create a supportive atmosphere for nursing students:

1. Establish a relationship and expectations. A good relationship with the manager or charge nurse on the unit helps establish a good student experience. Therefore, when a new group of student nurses comes to the floor, have one consistent contact meet and welcome them as a group. Take this opportunity to communicate the expectation that

- students have a valuable and positive experience
- any problems be brought to the manager's attention
- the door is open for feedback
- students are valued and honored

There have been times on our unit when students felt like they were an imposition and a hindrance to their mentors. Counseling the mentors helped improve the situation tremendously. Caught in the momentum of their work, preceptors were not aware that they were coming across as unavailable and unappreciative.

2. Educate the students. As the first group of students rotated through our unit, complaints from members of the nursing staff started piling up. The majority were territorial: "They're in our space," "I can't tape report when they're in there at 2:00," "They interrupt me to ask where another nurse is," etc.

To deal with the issue, the charge nurses got together to problem solve. They produced a one-page sheet for the students, called "Tips for a Great Nursing Experience." The sheet began with a sincere welcome: "We are very excited to have students on our unit and want to work together to make it a positive experience for all." It ended with, "We hope your experience was valuable. Please feel free to let us know how we can best work with you. We would love to hear your feedback."

Tips included the following:
- Try to avoid change of shift for data collection.

- Please vacate the conference room a half hour before end of shift so nurses can tape report.

- Feel free to ask the charge nurse for help if your nurse is busy (rather than asking other nurses).

- Chart at the chart rack or nearest hub. Put charts away when not using them.

- Give new orders to the unit secretary promptly.

Instructors provided students with the sheet upon arrival, and we never heard another complaint.

3. Educate all staff nurses. At staff meetings, I point out emphatically that students and new grads are not walking into the same world that current nurses found when they started. We need to demonstrate this fact to all parties involved and make sure that they understand and acknowledge this difference. Changes that are slow and incremental often go unnoticed (see human adaptability theory, Chapter 2). Here are a few examples I use for teaching:

- **The telephone.** Remember when you would let the telephone ring seven or eight times before hanging up? It was less than 10 years ago, but now that number has slowly gone down to three or four rings. Changes that are not noticeable and that happen over time are not obvious.

- **The frog parable.** If you put a frog into hot water, he jumps out immediately. If you put a frog into cool water and slowly turn up the temperature, the frog will boil to death. At no point will he jump out. *How hot is the water at your facility?* The temperature of the water that new grads are jumping into today is much hotter than it used to be.

- **Nursing.** Over the past ten years, there have been numerous incremental changes in the nurses' workload on the unit. There are many more drugs available, more patients with secondary and chronic illness, an increasingly obese patient population, and a decreasing length of stay.

The result of sharing this perspective has been an increase in compassion and understanding, with staff nurses reframing their attitudes and demonstrating more empathy. New nurses feel less judged and feel validated for the difficulties they are experiencing and report feeling a greater level of support.

4. Hold an annual roundtable with the managers from the hospital and instructors that have clinical rotations. At one of our roundtable discussions, we learned that students reported not feeling like the institution went out of its way for students. An all-day event, scheduled to kick off the year, remedied the problem.

With nurses scattered throughout the hospital, an event that brings all parties together for the purpose of validating, connecting, and imparting the values of that institution is prudent. It is an opportunity for CNOs and nursing leadership to increase their visibility and for managers to showcase their own departments.

5. Revise the curriculum. Education must address the culture and social construct of nursing. There should not be any "surprises" when new nurses hit the floor. An in-depth understanding of horizontal hostility will enable students not only to handle difficult situations but also to be catalysts for change. High-level communication and assertiveness skills should be taught and practiced. "Providing an educational forum on lateral violence for newly licensed nurses in orientation is essential for raising consciousness" (Griffin 2004).

All nurses, not just resident and student nurses, benefit from education on horizontal hostility. Staff need to know what nurse-to-nurse hostility is, as well as its effects and the solutions. To start getting the message out, consider distributing a fact sheet to employees (see Figure 5.1).

Figure 5.1　　　　　**Nurse-to-nurse hostility fact sheet**

What is nurse-to-nurse hostility?

Nurse-to-nurse hostility, also known as horizontal violence, colleague abuse, interpersonal conflict among coworkers, and workplace bullying, is a serious issue in the nursing profession that needs to be acknowledged and addressed.

Examples

1) Verbal hostility: insulting remarks, criticism, bickering, put-downs, shouting, talking behind a colleague's back, name-calling, intimidation, using a negative tone of voice, or withholding information from a colleague regarding a patient

2) Physical hostility: turning away, raising eyebrows, refusing to help, ignoring or obstructing the way of a colleague, intimidation using posture, hitting, assaulting, stabbing, or even shooting

Effects
- Feelings of: anxiety, fear, shock, anger, guilt, vulnerability, and humiliation
- Loss of self-confidence
- Lowered self-esteem
- Feeling threatened
- Developing stress-related illness
- Contemplating suicide

Solutions
At an organizational level:
- Adopt a zero-tolerance policy

Figure 5.1 | **Nurse-to-nurse hostility fact sheet (cont.)**

- Embrace a transformational leadership (with leaders who take a stand on issues, inspire, and have a positive vision)
- Develop a strong policy to deal with incidents of hostility, including a system of recordkeeping and accountability
- Develop institutional policies that are proactive, not reactive
- Develop a workable plan that gives managers the tools to act swiftly when an incident occurs
- Empower staff to speak without fear of reprisal

At an individual level:
- Gain control. Recognize that the aggressor is at fault—not you.
- Get help from your employer. Read your workplace policy on harassment or horizontal hostility to understand your options.
- Make an action plan. Seek advice from others with similar experiences, talk to your manager or counselor, and take advantage of employee assistance programs.
- Take action. Keep a detailed log of all incidents with names of witnesses. If your health is affected by these events, see your healthcare provider.
- Confront the aggressor. Make it clear that the behavior is offensive and must stop. Use the word "I" and specifically describe the behavior and how it made you feel.
- Make a formal written complain. Follow the grievance procedures provided by your organization or union.
- Take legal action. As a last resort, consider seeking expert legal advice.

Source: Jacoba Leiper, RN, MSN, lecturer at the University of North Carolina at Greensboro School of Nursing. Reprinted with permission.

6. Debrief, debrief, debrief! Make this a priority every day, not just at the end of the student's experience. Although course feedback has been in place for years, augmenting this feedback with the opportunity to share personal reflections from students' and new grads' experiences will benefit everyone. Optimally, debriefing should occur at every level—with the nurse, the manager, and the instructor.

One instructor who provided daily time for reflective practice said the following:

"It was difficult at first as no one wanted to appear vulnerable or share how they felt. So I started. I started with how inadequate and frustrated I felt covering all nine of them during a particular time when I was helping with a dressing change. Demonstrating my vulnerability seemed to be the key. It was as if suddenly I had given them permission to feel. After they started trusting me and each other, they began to open up.

For them, I am creating a very different scenario than I what got [as a student]: respect, dignity, and continuous learning. I encourage them to use each other as resources, which prevents them from putting others down."

When we stop to share our vulnerability, we acknowledge our humanness. There is a great deal of strength and solidarity that comes with realizing that no one is perfect, we all make mistakes, and we all feel vulnerable or afraid at times. A formal debriefing process offers nurses an opportunity to practice being authentically present in the workplace. Instead of immediately jumping to conclusions and sulking, we can speak our truth. From our authenticity comes our power.

When speaking our truth, we must begin our sentences with the most powerful word of all: **I**.

*"When you made that comment about the IV being dry for evening shift, **I** felt really picked on. **I** felt like you were putting me down."*

We are no longer victims when we speak our truth. Responding from our authentic self is an invitation for others to do the same. These conversations are the building blocks of a new culture.

*"Yes, **I** was frustrated because that's the third time this week **I** have come onto the shift and had to run and get a new IV. **I** guess **I** should have come to you personally instead of making an offhanded comment."*

Debriefing is an excellent opportunity to elicit emotions and role model healthy responses. These conversations represent the beginning of a new culture—a supportive culture where nurses feel confident and safe in expressing their feelings. There is an even greater opportunity for this culture to take hold if its roots are firmly established in nursing school.

Bringing horizontal hostility to light at nursing schools

Nursing educators are not immune to the pressures inherent in nursing. If you are in the nursing profession in any capacity, you have been asked to do more with less. Research shows that educators perceive their greatest stressor to be a heavy workload—more specifically, combined clinical and classroom teaching, as well as research (Goldenberg and Waddell 1990).

To say that horizontal hostility started in nursing school—or in any one arena, for that matter—would be to deny its cyclical nature. It "started" long ago in the subordinate origins of nursing, gathered momentum with a host of factors discussed in Section I, and now permeates every level of our profession. Because it is a part of the culture, no one in nursing is immune to its effects.

Every profession has a particular culture that is reinforced in school by its educators. If we are to change the culture, educators must be aware of and discuss the overt and covert ways that we disempower nurses. "Students are not encouraged from the start. There is more emphasis on judging than on assisting and supporting them" (Thomas 2004).

"No one in the class raised their hand, so I thought I would give it a try. That's the last time I do that. She put me down in front of everyone by saying, 'Now, you know better than that.' "

"I was in my fourth quarter, and I made a mistake. Right in front of the patient, the instructor put me down and pointed out my error. She did that to everyone. She could have taken us aside and saved some of our self-esteem."

See the problem

We are all the "culture carriers" of nursing. Our educational system is completely enmeshed in the culture of nursing and is not "the problem." It can be, however, a large part of the solution if we realize that it is one of the primary areas where nursing's subordinate position is reinforced (Roberts 1983).

Studies show that new nurses do not lack autonomy. When female nursing students were compared with female students from the schools of education, business, technology, and arts and sciences just prior to graduation, nurses scored higher on autonomy-related attitudes and behaviors (Boughn 1992). Nor do new nurses lack an understanding of their roles (Cook et al. 2003). Thus, autonomy and a sense of identity must diminish significantly *after* nurses are acculturated into the hospital environment.

Students are pivotal to solving the problem of horizontal hostility because they are not yet acculturated—with new eyes, they can see what we have accepted as normal. **If given the opportunity, students can recognize and articulate the practices that diminish them.**

Education, therefore, needs to be designed to "see through" the consciousness that is and will be imposed on students by the dominant group (Freshwater 2000). Learning must emancipate students. A transformative learning model based on critical theory, which addresses through self-reflection the fact that many barriers to empowerment are self-imposed, can help accomplish this goal (Freshwater 2000). Debriefing sessions can be held in small groups and the key points of each group shared with the class. Any exercise or intervention that stimulates understanding through reflection is a winner.

Create a narrative community

A useful technique for facilitating reflection is "narrative community," a concept created by Mary Schoessler, RN, MS, EdD, for newly graduated nurses. The thinking behind the technique is that stories are a powerful medium that give voice to who you are. The concept stresses that new graduates need to process both their triumphs and their failures in order to cope with their emotional responses and to use the experiences as sources of learning and growth

(Schoessler 2005). Narrative community seeks to create the safe space needed to discuss difficult subjects and bring meaning and understanding to the nursing practice.

When creating a narrative community, an individual the group trusts should facilitate the sessions. This person must listen and reflect on each participant's experience, suggest a context for the experience, and highlight the reasons for hope. Schoessler suggests bringing groups of 10–15 nurses together on a regular basis and setting down some important ground rules for successful group work. Ground rules may include listening carefully to understand and to learn, sharing stories, using "I" language, and keeping all stories told in the group confidential.

New resident nurses

"Nurse administrators and staff nurses often carry on where the faculty leave off. When new graduates hit the workplace, their idealism may be mocked and their short-comings magnified."

—*Thomas (2004)*

New graduates report that stress and job conflict are the top problems in their first year of employment (McKenna et al. 2003). Nurses who feel a lack of support and are frustrated due to intrinsic and extrinsic factors (see Chapter 3) take out those feelings on new grads, and the vicious cycle of hostility continues. Thus, the first line of defense in winning the battle against horizontal hostility is nurse educators; the second line of defense is nurse administrators and staff nurses.

The strategies mentioned earlier in the chapter focused on educating new nurses, educators, and staff nurses about the realities of the floor. In addition to those interventions, new resident nurses also can benefit from the following:

1. Preceptor feedback. At the end of orientation, have the new resident nurse fill out a questionnaire about his or her preceptor. This feedback, presented constructively, provides mentors with specific and detailed information. This communication is critical: It stops the "down only" flow of information and evens the playing field. It also sets the tone for reciprocity, as well as for professional and collegial relationships. Two-way communication debunks the myth that any of us are perfect. By soliciting it, managers and educators send the message that they care about the experiences of new nurses.

2. One-on-one time. It is a well-known fact that bonding is critical and that the new grad's experience in the first two months may predict how many years she or he will stay. We have not acknowledged, however, that we have adapted to a faster work pace and have less time for bonding. Therefore, we must make an additional effort to

- relieve a nurse and her preceptor so that they can have lunch together and time to debrief

- allow every staff member to share a meal with the new resident nurse every day for the first two weeks (fosters assimilation into the group by creating belonging)

- decrease a precepting nurse's usual workload

3. Reflective practice. "Reflective practice through clinical supervision is a potential space for transformatory learning to take place, to bring to awareness the conflicts between the inner and the outer dialogue, and issues of inequality and power distance that are often suppressed within the work setting" (Freshwater 2000). Encouraging new nurses to stop and reflect on their day prevents mixed emotions from building up and leading to anger. It also helps to clarify issues so that they can be addressed constructively.

Although debriefing is usually a group process, reflection can also occur individually through journaling or peer-to-peer time. Sharing our experiences is a powerful way to connect and to make sense of our nursing culture. This introspection builds confidence and autonomy and helps us form the strong emotional bonds that are so critical to group cohesion.

4. Education and cognitive rehearsal. Research shows that educating new nurses about horizontal hostility allows them "to depersonalize it, thus allowing them to ask questions and continue to learn" (Griffin 2004). Learning is severely compromised when new nurses feel that it is not safe to ask questions in the work environment (Sternberg and Horvath 1998).

In 2004, the *Journal of Continuing Education in Nursing* published an exploratory study on the effects of using cognitive skills as a shield from lateral violence. In the study, a group of 26 new nurses were taught cognitive responses that increased their interpersonal skills and enabled them to confront their offenders. After classroom instruction in which nurses practiced confrontation skills, new nurses were provided with two cards. The first card (Figure 5.2) listed the universally accepted behavioral expectations for any given group of professionals. The second card (Figure 5.3) listed appropriate verbal responses to the most common forms of lateral violence and was attached to the nurses' identification badges so that, in the event of a conflict, the nurses could reference the information immediately (Griffin 2004).

Figure 5.2

Expected behaviors of those who call themselves professionals

- Accept one's fair share of the workload.
- Respect the privacy of others.
- Be cooperative with regard to the shared physical working conditions (e.g., light, temperature, noise).
- Be willing to help when help is requested.
- Keep confidences.
- Work cooperatively, despite feelings of dislike.
- Don't denigrate to superiors (e.g., speak negatively about, have a pet name for).
- Do address coworkers by their first name, and ask for help and advice when necessary.
- Look coworkers in the eye when having a conversation.
- Don't be overly inquisitive about each others' lives.
- Do repay debts, favors, and compliments, no matter how small.
- Don't engage in conversation about a coworker with another coworker.
- Stand up for the "absent member" in a conversation when he or she is not present.
- Don't criticize publicly.

Adapted from Arglye & Henderson, 1985; Chaska, 2001. SLACK Incorporated and
The Journal of Continuing Education in Nursing. *Reprinted with permission.*

Figure 5.3

Cueing cards attached to identification badge

SIDE 1

Nonverbal innuendo (raising of eyebrows, face-making).

- I sense (I see from your facial expression) that there may be something you wanted to say to me. It's okay to speak directly to me.

Verbal affront (covert or overt, snide remarks, lack of openness, abrupt responses).

- The individuals I learn the most from are clearer in their directions and feedback. Is there some way we can structure this type of situation?

Undermining activities (turning away, being unavailable).

- When something happens that is "different" or "contrary" to what I thought or understood, it leaves me with questions. Help me understand how this situation may have happened.

Withholding information (practice or patient).

- It is my understanding that there was (is) more information available regarding the situation, and I believe if I had known that (more), it would (will) affect how I learn.

Sabotage (deliberately setting up a negative situation).

- There is more to this situation than meets the eye. Could "you and I" (whatever, whoever) meet in private and explore what happened?

SIDE 2

Infighting (bickering with peers). Nothing is more unprofessional than a contentious discussion in a nonprivate place. Always avoid.

- This is not the time or the place. Please stop (physically walk away or move to a neutral spot).

Scapegoating (attributing all that goes wrong to one individual). Rarely is one individual, one incident, or one situation the cause for all that goes wrong. Scapegoating is an easy route to travel, but it rarely solves problems.

- I don't think that's the right connection.

Backstabbing (complaining to others about an individual and not speaking directly to that individual).

- I don't feel right talking about him/her/the situation when I wasn't there or don't know the facts. Have you spoken to him/her?

Failure to respect privacy.

- It bothers me to talk about that without his/her/their permission.
- I only overheard that. It shouldn't be repeated.

Broken confidences.

- Wasn't that said in confidence?
- That sounds like information that should remain confidential.
- He/she asked me to keep that confidential.

Single card attached to ID

- Accept one's fair share of the workload.
- Respect the privacy of others.
- Be cooperative with regard to the shared physical working conditions (e.g., light, temperature, noise).
- Be willing to help when requested.
- Keep confidences.
- Work cooperatively despite feelings of dislike.
- Don't denigrate to superiors (e.g., speak negatively about, have a pet name for).
- Do address coworkers by their first name, and ask for help and advice when necessary.
- Look coworkers in the eye when having a conversation.
- Don't be overly inquisitive about each others' lives.
- Do repay debts, favors, and compliments, no matter how small.
- Don't engage in conversation about a coworker with another coworker.
- Stand-up for the "absent member" in a conversation when he/she is not present.
- Don't criticize publicly.

SLACK Incorporated and The Journal of Continuing Education in Nursing. *Reprinted with permission.*

After a year, all participants were evaluated. "There appeared to be one distinctive outcome among those confronted. The laterally violent behavior stopped" (Griffin 2004). The nurses reported that they did not need to look at the cards at the time of the event because they understood the information on them and remembered what they had learned in the lecture and interactive sessions. "Knowledge of lateral violence and a behavioral action to stop it (cognitive rehearsal)" empowered nurses to successfully confront abusive nurses (Griffin 2004).

5. Innovative programs. Nursing administrators all over the country are leading efforts to design programs focused on supporting new graduates.

When Moses Cone Hospital in Greensboro, NC, realized that it was losing a significant number of new grads within the first two years, they developed the Graduate Advancement Program (GAP) to better assimilate new nurses into the profession. The program complements the hospital's departmental orientation and provides graduates with a yearlong mentorship with an experienced leader, who supports the student and helps him or her to build confidence and competency. New nurses are placed in cohorts of ten with a mentor with whom they meet once a month for a year after the initial one-week orientation. The group is a safe place for reflective practice, and the new nurses' stories strengthen the bonds between them as they share their first death or an experience with a senior nurse that was degrading. For example, the cohorts meet with physicians to discuss openly the "things that scare them." With almost no experience in dealing with physicians prior to their hospital experience, new nurses have a lot of questions, and the time with the physicians helps them decrease anxiety and build relationships.

According to Joan Wessman, RN, MS, CNO, of Moses Cone, having this critical infrastructure in place to support new grads played a major role in boosting the retention rate from 64% to an impressive 97%. Both administration and new graduates benefit from the GAP program, Wessman said. "These nurses have grown in confidence and in an understanding of the role [of a nurse]. We learned that we didn't know this group as much as we should . . . [and] that meaningful relationships are important," she said.

Summary

Strategies designed to improve the experience of nursing students and resident nurses have one common denominator: They help form meaningful relationships. To new nurses, this connection is vital because such relationships provide a safe place to exercise their voices. Our voice is our power. Every opportunity to express ourselves increases self-esteem.

New nurses need the freedom, confidence, and permission to verbalize concerns. Whether by using reflective practice, one-on-one time, or a retention program, they must find the support they need because it allows them to speak their truth. By doing so, they build and nourish their personal power.

Feedback from new nurses is critical, as they can best see the negative practices that our nursing culture has normalized. But nothing will change until we can openly discuss and identify the ways in which we deny empowerment. "Liberation from oppression is accomplished through a process in which education and insight into the cycle leads to connection, support, and improved self-esteem among oppressed people" (Freire 1990).

Horizontal hostility's roots have been firmly set in an uneven power struggle. The way to break out of the cycle of oppression is to illuminate the behaviors and raise our self-esteem (Roberts 1983). When self-esteem is low, individuals are powerless to change their situation (Randle 2003). Thus, the very act of taking back our power raises our self-esteem.

The key to breaking out of this cycle, therefore, is empowerment. "Empowerment is a helping process whereby groups or individuals are enabled to change a situation, given skills, resources, opportunities, and authority to do so. It is a partnership which respects and values self and others" (Rodwell 1996). This partnership between teachers and students is the new archetype we must create.

Recommended reading

Crosscurrents: Against cultural narration in nursing. *Journal of Advanced Nursing.*
　By Dawn Freshwater

Teaching cognitive rehearsal as a shield for lateral violence: An intervention for newly licensed nurses. *Journal of Continuing Education in Nursing.*
　By M. Griffin

Bibliography

Boughn, S. 1992. Nursing students rank high in autonomy at the exit level. *Journal of Nursing Education* 31(2): 58–64.

Cook, T., et al. 2003. Beginning students' definitions of nursing: an inductive framework of professional identity. *Journal of Nurse Educators* 42(7):311-317.

Davey, L. 2002. Nurses eating nurses: The caring profession which fails to nurture its own. *Contemporary Nurse* 13(2–3): 192–197.

Freire, P. 1990. *Pedagogy of the Oppressed.* New York: Continuum International Publishing.

Freshwater, D. 2000. Crosscurrents: against cultural narration in nursing. *Journal of Advanced Nursing* 32(2).

Goldenberg, D., and J. Waddell. 1990. Occupational stress and coping strategies among female baccalaureate nursing faculty. *Journal of Advanced Nursing* 15(5): 531–43.

Griffin, M. 2004. Teaching Cognitive Rehearsal as a shield for lateral violence: an intervention for newly licensed nurses. *The Journal of Continuing Education in Nursing* 35(6).

Keuter, K., et al. 2000. Nurses' job satisfaction and organizational climate in a dynamic work environment. *Applied Nursing Research* 13(1): 46–49.

McKenna, B., et al. 2003. Horizontal violence: Experiences of registered nurses in their first year of practice. *Journal of Advanced Nursing* 42(1): 90–96.

Moses Cone Health System. New Graduates: Graduate Advancement Program. *www.mosescone.com/body.cfm?id=540*.

Randle, J. 2003. Bullying in the nursing profession. *Journal of Advanced Nursing* 43(4): 395–401.

Roberts, S. 1983. Oppressed group behavior: implications for nursing. *Advances in Nursing Science* 5(4): 21–30.

Rodwell, C. 1996. An analysis of the concept of empowerment. *Journal of Advanced Nursing* 23(2): 305–313.

Schoessler, Mary. 2005. *Narrative Community for newly graduated nurses.* Self-published.

Sternberg, R., and J. Horvath. 1998. *Tacit Knowledge in Professional Practice.* Mahwah, NJ: Lawrence Erlbaum Associates.

Thomas, S. 2004. *Transforming Nurses' Stress and Anger: Steps Toward Healing.* New York: Springer Publishing Company.

Viverais-Dresler, G., and M. Kutschke. 2001. RN students' ratings and opinions related to the importance of certain clinical teacher behaviors. *Journal of Continuing Education in Nursing* 32(6): 274–82.

CHAPTER SIX

Managerial response

"Managers are the culture carriers of the organization."

—Farrell (2005)

In the movie, *What the Bleep Do We Know?!,* there is a scene set in the late 1400s on the coast of what is now the United States. Three tall ships have arrived at the harbor, but the villagers cannot see them because they have no frame of reference. Never in their wildest dreams would they have imagined a boat could be so huge. And so they can't see the ships. The shaman of the village stares out over the water. He has noticed that the wave pattern is different and tunes in to a strange sound. Eventually, after days and days of staring over the water, the shaman can see the ships.

And so it is with nursing leaders. Like the shaman, we must be observant and notice the small changes in our environment that reflect a larger behavior—one that is so emotionally engaging that we cannot see the profound effect it has on the work environment. As leaders, success in eliminating horizontal hostility will depend on 1) our ability to see the problem, 2) our communication network, and 3) our response.

Awareness: Ability to see the problem

Researchers often use the word "insidious" to describe horizontal hostility because it has existed as an undercurrent of our profession for years. Not only is the behavior hidden, but the costs are hidden as well, *as the financial impact lags behind the actual events*. And when its destruction becomes obvious, it is usually too late—a high turnover results not only in a mass exodus of staff but also in a crucial break in the unit's knowledge base.

Indications of horizontal hostility

The following are often indications of horizontal hostility:

- **Poor employee satisfaction scores.** Satisfaction surveys differ in content from facility to facility, but there are usually some similarities. The scores you should be most interested in are "intent to leave," "sense of belonging," "meaningful work," "morale of self," and "morale of others." One of the telltale signs of horizontal hostility on the unit is when staff rate "others' morale" significantly lower than their own. This is because staff who hear a lot of gossip and negativity naturally conclude that their peers' morale is much lower than their own.

- **High turnover rates.** This is an obvious indicator of horizontal hostility. Staff who feel that they belong will clearly want to stay—and vice versa. The key to preventing a mass exodus is to follow up with an employee the moment you get the "heads up" that he or she may be leaving. Timely follow-up is crucial at this point, as the staff member's reasons for leaving may alert you to a larger problem—a problem that, if continued, could lead to more resignations.

On my unit, it was not until after a staff member left the floor for another unit that I discovered the true cause of her transfer: Two employees who ate together, covered each other's patients, and took breaks together had formed an impenetrable "clique."

- **Dueling units, dueling shifts.** I was in charge of two floors. For the first six months in my new position as manager, I heard numerous complaints as staff whined they didn't want to float "there." In between the lines was the message that both floors felt that "our floor is harder than yours."

Weary of the lack of respect between shifts, I asked the charge nurses to switch shifts for a week. After only one day, the charge nurses asked to return to their normal floors, but we held firm to the original plan. The charge nurses quickly learned that the floors each had different challenges of their own, and a new respect for those challenges emerged. I never heard another complaint.

The same plan worked beautifully when shift-to-shift complaints starting filtering through. "Walking in each other's shoes" was a powerful tool to help staff understand that different floors and different shifts each have their own unique set of challenges.

- **Presence of cliques.** A clique can include anywhere from two people to an entire floor. Members of the night shift often form a particularly tight group because they depend so much on each other. Years of working together result in a finely choreographed ballet as the nurses cover each other and the unit.

Signs of a clique include
  - staff who consistently refuse to work with someone or prefer to work with someone specific
  - a staff member who always volunteers to float

- exclusive meal breaks—i.e., same people, all the time, others not invited
- refusal to help, which results in nurses feeling like they are "sinking" due to a lack of teamwork
- staff who change assignments or the schedule to work (or not work) with certain people

• **Incident reports.** Be aware if these reports are always filled out by the same person or are on the same person. A nurse consistently writing up her peers may have a "witch-hunt" mentality. These nurses are usually very passive-aggressive—they would never directly tell another nurse about a problem. This fact is usually indicative of a much larger issue. For example, the nurse may lack the confrontation skills necessary to handle the situation, or there may be a group effort to force a particular staff member to leave.

• **Absenteeism.** There are many physical and psychological signs and symptoms of horizontal hostility. Frequent illness is often an indicator of a larger problem. Staff who are particularly vulnerable are those who lack support systems and usually have issues they are dealing with at home as well. Run an absentee report, and check in with staff who have more than four absences per year.

• **Behavior clues.** Employees who are victims of or witnesses to horizontal hostility may withdraw and shut down as a way of protecting themselves (Farrell 2005). Horizontal hostility needs silent witnesses in order to exist, so pull these employees aside and provide them with a safe climate in which they can express their feelings. "Nurses who are 'silent' in the workplace do not believe that their true self is being expressed, [nor do they feel] professionally independent and valued as a nurse" (DeMarco et al. 2005).

Ways to assess whether horizontal hostility is a problem on your unit

The following are methods for evaluating staff and assessing the problem of horizontal hostility on your unit. If after assessing these areas you feel that your team is in good shape, continue to monitor the environment:

- **Use questionnaires to assess the cohesiveness, productivity, and psychological safety of your team.** Questionnaires can elicit a wealth of information. Such questionnaires do not need to be extensive, and they should always end with an open-ended question. They often help with assessment because although we might *think* that we have a good handle on the climate, we often do not. Because horizontal hostility is insidious, because we have an intense workload, and because this behavior has been accepted as normal for years, it often exists outside of the realm of our awareness. Simply "checking in" with managers or staff is empowering because it sends the message that you want to know the truth.

"When questionnaires were returned, we found that nurses scored very high on feeling supported and safe. But then there were questions asking, 'Can you approach a coworker about an error?' and 'Can you talk to your peers about a rumor you heard about yourself?,' and the answers were at the other end of the spectrum. It was very enlightening to show staff the results and ask, 'What's wrong with this picture?' 'Why can't you talk to your peers if you feel safe and supported?'"

"We found that 52% of staff had participated in a negative discussion about a coworker in the last month . . . gossip was the most prevalent overt cue and the biggest surprise was that silence, then sarcasm, were the most prevalent covert cues."

- **Use nominal group technique.** In this process, a question or problem is written down on the board and team members write down their ideas/solutions. Then each person reads one idea off of his or her list, with no discussion, and the ideas are all listed for everyone to see. Team members assign points to the most important idea/solution, and the votes are tallied on a flip chart (Scholtes 1988).

Nominal group technique is an effective tool not only with new groups but also with any staff who are stuck on a controversial issue. It facilitates input with a low level of interaction. At one facility, when managers were extremely disgruntled among themselves but would not take their issues to administration, nominal group technique was used with great success to validate concerns and develop constructive solutions.

Any intervention that encourages nurses to speak freely will not only give leaders the information they need to design interventions, but will make a statement. The questions become the expectations, and the answers will become expressions of power and enlightenment.

Clues that horizontal hostility exists can be direct or indirect. Increased complaints of poor patient care, rumors about staff leaving, negative employee satisfaction scores, and absenteeism are direct. Indirect effects include sarcasm, manipulation of assignments and schedules, disgruntled employees who are always negative, and gossip that circulates 24 hours a day. The only way to keep your finger on the pulse of hostility on your unit is to form strong relationships with key staff and maintain an open communication network.

Consider distributing one or both of the following questionnaires to gauge staff feelings and to assess the prevalence of horizontal hostility at your facility.

Figure 6.1	Sample questionnaire

1 = Agree strongly
2 = Agree
3 = Not certain
4 = Disagree
5 = Disagree strongly

	1	2	3	4	5
I am respected by my peers.	1	2	3	4	5
I feel supported by my peers.	1	2	3	4	5
My work group is a safe environment in which to express my opinions.	1	2	3	4	5
If I have a problem with any member of this group, I feel good about talking to that person directly.	1	2	3	4	5
My peers respect my opinion.	1	2	3	4	5
I have good working relationships with all team members.	1	2	3	4	5
In the past month, I have not participated in any discussion about a team member who is not present.	1	2	3	4	5

What I like the most about this team is _____

What I need more from this group is _____

| Figure 6.2 | Verbal abuse survey |

Please answer the following questions by circling (1) low, (2) medium, or (3) high.

1. The amount of self-esteem I normally have is: 1   2   3
2. The amount of assertiveness I normally demonstrate is: 1   2   3
3. I perceive my level of competence in nursing practice to be: 1   2   3
4. The amount of control I believe I have over my own nursing
   practice in my current position is: 1   2   3

Please circle your chosen answer.

1. In your work experience as an RN, have you ever had an experience
   in which you have been verbally abused?   Yes   No
2. How would you rate your handling of verbally abusive situations?
        Poor   Fair   Good   Very Good
3. Which of the following best describes your feelings following a verbally abusive incident? Circle all
   that apply.
        Angry   Confused   Determined to problem solve   Embarrassed
        Fearful   Harassed Hostile   Powerless   Other
4. Did the verbal abuse occur during or immediately after a high-stress situation
   for either you or the abuser?   Yes   No
5. During one month's time, of approximately how many abusive statements
   (from all sources) are you the recipient?   0–5   6–10   11–15   16–20   more than 20
6. Have you ever taken assertiveness training classes?
        Yes   No   If yes, when? _____

Based on your experience with verbal abuse, do you believe

1. the incident had a negative effect on your morale?
        Yes   No   Comments _____
2. the incident caused a decrease in your level of productivity for a period of time?
        Yes   No   Comments _____
3. such incidents lead to an increase in errors?
        Yes   No   Comments _____
4. the incident's effect contributed to an increased workload for your coworkers for a period of time?
        Yes   No   Comments _____
5. the incident influenced your delivery of nursing care for a period of time?
        Yes   No   Comments _____

Source: Helen Cox, RN, EdD, and Laura Sofield, RN, MSN. Revised and adapted with permission.

Communication

"Even among friends, starting a conversation can take courage. But conversation also gives us courage. Thinking together, deciding what actions to take, more of us become bold. As we learn from each other's experiences and interpretations, we see the issue in richer detail. We understand more of the dynamics that have created it. With this clarity, we know what actions to take and where we might have the most influence."

—Wheatley (2002)

A manager should focus on assessing the unit's communication network. Can anyone bring up *any subject* at staff meetings? In private? Because we cannot possibly be on the unit 24 hours a day, managers need to create a strong communication network. Creating an environment of open communication where staff feel psychologically safe is critical. Such an atmosphere invites staff to talk about difficult subjects and often allows us to get a "heads up" before a behavior escalates.

The mob squad

It was only my third week as a new manager. As I was leaving for the day, the charge nurse tentatively approached me.

"I thought you might want to know that the night shift is really bad-mouthing you," she said. I asked her to tell me more. "Susan said you can't change the schedule because it was written into the union contract, and Deb and Megan are really angry. They said you're not touching their schedules." I thanked her for sharing the information.

I arrived at 6:30 the next day and asked to see Susan, Deb, and Megan in the charge nurse's office. To say they were surprised would be a gross understatement. To their shock, I restated the gossip that I had heard. I explained that although I had no inten-tion of changing the schedule, there would need to be some shifting of the current sched-ule due to new grads—and that the old union contract no longer held.

Emphatically, I told the nurses that I would have no chance of being a successful manager without their support—as long as they "talked me down" behind my back, I was doomed. I relayed my expectation that they come to me directly with any problems or concerns and assured them that I was confident that we could solve any problem—together.

"Negative emotions will just kill a unit by demoralizing staff," I said. "They create a toxic atmosphere that no one would want to work in."

Slowly, my words diffused their anger. I realized that fear was at the root of their emo-tional outburst and that I needed the cohesiveness of this group.

"My plan is to have self-scheduling as much as possible, and because night shift seems like such a strong group, maybe you would be willing to take over the responsibility for your schedule. I can give you the new grad's FTE."

They agreed. When the new schedule was finished, I had to smile at the new patterns. For the next five years, the night shift nurses put out their schedule on their own.

In systems theory, this would be analogous to an "open system"—an environment where staff can speak their truth without fear of retribution. Role modeling is a critical way of educating staff and creating and maintaining an open system. If you hear a rumor and go directly to that staff member to check it out, your staff will do the same with you.

Managers can build communication skills that are characteristic of an open system by promoting the following:

- Charge nurse development
- Inservices on assertiveness, confrontation skills, and conflict resolution
- Role modeling
- Performance evaluations

Charge nurse development: Leadership skills

Getting charge nurses or key people on board allows you to communicate zero tolerance for horizontal hostility. Horizontal hostility needs secrecy, shame, and silent witnesses to continue, and all of these ingredients exist in a closed system (Namie and Namie 2000). Changing to an open system requires staff involvement and a strong communication network that imparts a new set of values and expectations.

Charge nurse retreat

A retreat for charge nurses is an invaluable tool in building cohesiveness and leadership abilities. In effect, a charge nurse retreat is an essential "time out." Stopping to acknowledge and appreciate each other is priceless. Before the retreat, nurses on our unit felt an unrealistic pressure to be perfect and feared failure. But after nurses shared their own individual struggles with each other, they realized that "we are all in the same boat." Charge nurses stopped judging themselves and each other so harshly. The time, attention, and education devoted to the charge nurses helped improve unit cohesion dramatically.

Our most recent retreat provided an education program focused on building leadership skills. Holding staff accountable was a top priority at our facility, but charge nurses often lacked the skills to do so, so people were "getting away with things."

"Go ahead," I would challenge them as we went around the table. "Give me your toughest scene; give me your worst confrontation." Then we would role-play the conflicts that were giving them such a challenge and were taking away their power. Armed with new scripts, the charge nurses went back to the unit and began holding staff accountable for their actions.

Proudly, the night charge nurse approached me the day after we returned from our skills workshop and said, "I did it! For years I have tolerated Terri's incomplete medication records, and last night I approached her with the problem it was causing and the expectation. I did it!" she said, beaming with pride. "And I thought it would take me three months to get up the courage."

Unit philosophy

At the retreat, the charge nurses all stated what they valued the most about nursing. Together they came up with a "Unit Philosophy," which they then asked all staff to sign. As manager, I explained to the staff that this unit philosophy was a product of all of the charge nurses getting together and sharing their values and beliefs, but now we needed their input.

After the philosophy was finalized, employees had only three choices: sign it, edit it and then sign it, or transfer out of the department. No one could live in the gray zone any longer. This posted document was a tangible reminder that everyone was, literally, on the same page. The following are some of the philosophy's key points:

- There will be a zero tolerance for gossip and negativity on the unit.

- We respect each other. Therefore, it is the expectation that any problems will be addressed in private with the person(s) involved.

- We recognize that, in order to create a healing environment for our patients, we must create it with each other first.

- We pledge to provide the highest quality of care by demonstrating excellent clinical competence.

A unit philosophy is a powerful way to unite staff. The mission, vision, and values of the hospital are often too vague, and staff have no direct input into their conception—therefore, there is no buy-in. Creating a unit philosophy empowers staff by giving them responsibility for their own work environment. It requires that staff answer the question, *"What do you value and what do you believe?"*

A new belief system

Slowly, we altered the belief system of the unit. Through education and mentoring, first the charge nurses and then the staff came to believe the following:

- There is enough for everyone.
- There are things we can control and things we can't.
- Nobody is perfect.
- Every single nurse on this floor has something special to offer. If you can't see it, look harder.
- Everyone has his or her own story. Don't make up one before you listen to theirs.
- Compassion and kindness go much further than judgment and blame.
- You won't melt or die by confronting someone with the truth.
- Our greatest strength is the relationships we have with each other.
- Negativity poisons the work atmosphere for everyone.
- We are all in the same boat. Climb in.
- We are only as strong as our weakest link.

- It is my responsibility to take care of myself and to verbalize my concerns.
- If I have a problem with someone, I will talk to him or her in private.

Individual action plans

One of the hallmarks of our charge nurse retreats became individual action plans. With the help of the leadership cards and a peer, staff would select the three areas in which they excelled, as well as the three areas they most wanted to improve. In addition, prior to the retreat, I asked the staff nurses to fill out a form giving feedback to each charge nurse (see Figure 6.3).

The responses were an eye opener to all. Staff nurses had never been asked for feedback, and those in charge nurse positions had never received it from staff. Soliciting this feedback sent a strong message to staff that the charge nurses were striving to improve and needed staff input to do so. Without the opportunity to give feedback, problems may have festered, ultimately resulting in hostile behaviors.

After reviewing the feedback responses and the selected leadership cards the charge nurses had chosen, we worked on detailed individual action plans for improvement. The action plans clearly listed the area on which the charge nurses most wanted to focus, specific steps to achieve the goal, a realistic time frame, and a way to measure success. These plans were kept in a binder in my office and referenced at performance evaluations and whenever possible.

Figure 6.3	Charge nurse assessment tool

Person requesting feedback _____

Circle your relationship to the person requesting feedback:

Self	Peer	Manager	I report to this person

Please rate the person on the following.

1 = poor	2 = fair	3 = good	4 = very good	5 = excellent

Quality care

1. Ensures the highest quality care and service for each person served.	1	2	3	4	5
2. Implements and monitors quality and patient standards.	1	2	3	4	5
3. Fosters a culture of non-blame for mistakes.	1	2	3	4	5
4. Points a finger at the solution instead of at people.	1	2	3	4	5
5. Applies win/win solutions to meet department and organizational goals.	1	2	3	4	5

Managing resources

6. Schedules staff in an efficient way.	1	2	3	4	5
7. Plans work fairly and efficiently (post-ops).	1	2	3	4	5
8. Is available as a resource to troubleshoot problems.	1	2	3	4	5
9. Rounds frequently with staff to assess needs.	1	2	3	4	5
10. Devises strategies to improve teamwork.	1	2	3	4	5
11. Is a dependable resource to staff: willing to step in when there are patient care needs and able to identify them when needed.	1	2	3	4	5

Figure 6.3	Charge nurse assessment tool (cont.)

Effective relationships

12. Consistently maintains a professional demeanor.	1	2	3	4	5
13. Maintains a positive attitude and fosters solutions.	1	2	3	4	5
14. Delivers feedback in a way that improves performance.	1	2	3	4	5
15. Receives feedback in a way that improves performance.	1	2	3	4	5
16. Demonstrates respectful listening.	1	2	3	4	5
17. Genuinely cares for others.	1	2	3	4	5
18. Observes and reflects on his or her own behavior.	1	2	3	4	5

Leadership

19. Consistently models Service Excellence commitments.	1	2	3	4	5
20. Is a patient advocate.	1	2	3	4	5
21. Actively builds relationships among staff, between departments, and with physicians.	1	2	3	4	5
22. Fosters a positive work environment.	1	2	3	4	5
23. Is easy to approach.	1	2	3	4	5
24. Acknowledges staff for a job well done.	1	2	3	4	5
25. Maintains a high sense of integrity.	1	2	3	4	5

What I appreciate the most about this charge nurse is _____

_____

_____

What I would really like to see more of is

_____

_____

Inservices on assertiveness and confrontation skills

The most effective classes are those that are attended by staff who work on the same shift. To accomplish this, I arranged for a series of crucial-conversation workshops from our Employee Learning Department and had members of every shift come in two hours early to attend the workshops. Instead of making these sessions mandatory, I explained the importance of addressing each shift's issues in the staff meetings and then asked for anyone who could not make the meeting to please let me know.

The essence of the course was that failure to speak your truth about issues—directly to the people involved—always ends up in either silence or hostility, and that neither is a healthy option. In this constructive atmosphere, staff began to share what bothered them, and then they learned the skills necessary to hold crucial conversations.

Staff reported that the workshops were extremely helpful and allowed them to verbalize repressed feelings. It was clear from the conversations in class that staff had not realized the impact that their failure to communicate had on others—and on themselves. After the first class, one of the nurses burst into my office.

"I did it!" she said, proudly. "After fifteen years I finally told Lydia how her negative comments bothered me. I feel like my blood pressure just dropped by 20!"

Now she is shaking and her eyes are filled with tears. "Why did it take me fifteen years to tell her that?!"

And then there was Andrea. All week long (before the workshop), she ruminated about an incident that really bothered her: She had walked up to Judy, who had immediately turned away from her, leaving her feeling rejected. Andrea wondered constantly about what she could have done to offend her. It affected her mood. It affected her mental clarity. And it affected her performance. Therefore, it affected all of us. Finally, after the crucial-conversation workshop, she was able to confront Judy.

"I felt like you didn't like something I said when you turned around and walked away so quickly without saying anything. That's the second time you've done that."

"I'm glad you checked that out," Judy replied. *"It wasn't anything you said or did. I was just preoccupied with wanting to get into my confused patient's room as quickly as I could after report because I was worried about him."*

In another case, a charge nurse decided to stop wallowing in her usual guilt about not being able to make her staff nurse's day go better. She went directly to the staff nurse to take care of the problem.

Charge nurse: "I feel very badly about your day. Was there anything I could have done to help that I overlooked?"

Staff nurse: "No, but it means a lot to me that you asked. I get so caught up . . ."

Charge nurse: "Yes, I see that, but it makes me frustrated because I end up feeling useless—helpless, even."

Staff nurse: "On second thought, maybe you could remind me to take a deep breath. That would help me slow down enough to give you some specific tasks that would lighten my load."

Unfortunately, not all nurses are holding these conversations. **Instead, they are holding rejection, fear, and all the feelings that cascade forth when we fail to understand a situation.** Typically, an angry nurse who sulks for the entire shift—and then projects her misery on everyone else—needs to learn healthy communication skills. Verbalizing our emotions is a lesson in empowerment. As mentioned in Section I, many nurses have a passive-aggressive style of communication, which means that they learned early on in life to not say anything that might upset someone. It takes courage for staff who have been disempowered for years to even use the word "I," let alone to verbalize their feelings, but doing so can lead to a greater feeling of self-respect.

Hierarchy of voice

There is a hierarchy of voice that I use to encourage nurses' self-esteem. It is a "hierarchy" because each step results in greater empowerment. In performance evaluations, I share the following list and ask staff to pick ten meaningful actions that they would like to perform to increase their self-esteem. Staff then label their choices from one to ten (easiest to hardest). Addressing specific behaviors that are a challenge to a nurse stimulates meaningful conversations about that individual's stumbling blocks to empowerment and self-esteem. I point out that each of the following actions incrementally builds self-esteem, respect, and autonomy:

- Introduce yourself to patients with a firm handshake.
- Use "Nurse" or "RN" when introducing yourself to patients and their families.
- Educate each patient about your role in his or her plan of care every day.
- Don't apologize when calling a physician.

- Use the progress notes for communicating any areas of concern to physicians.
- Invite a new nurse or nursing assistant to eat lunch with you.
- Shake hands with and introduce yourself to all new physicians and staff.
- Expect physicians with whom you work daily to know your name. Remind them, if necessary.
- If you witness an abusive interaction, report it to the manager.
- Volunteer to represent your organization at community events.
- Use reflective practice to recognize your skills and attributes.
- Compliment a coworker every shift; recognize his or her skills and attributes.
- Always use "I" when approaching another peer with a problem.
- Speak your truth. Verbalize your feelings.
- Bring concerns that cannot be resolved to the manager's attention.
- Participate in shared governance.
- Refuse to participate in gossip.
- Don't sit by and say or do nothing while someone else is being talked about negatively. State that the issue should be brought up with the person involved, and then leave.
- Identify a problem AND its solution for the unit. Then share it with everyone.
- Write an article or editorial for a newsletter.
- Make a presentation at physician rounds.
- Participate in regional nursing conferences and events.
- Speak at your nursing specialty's national conference.

Growing pains, growing skills

A new volunteer at the front desk was causing a lot of disruption. He was loud and talkative. He was annoying. Diane, the charge nurse, asked me if I could say something to him.

"Why don't you?" I responded.

"No way," she said stubbornly. "I just don't feel comfortable."

"Let me rephrase the question." I said. "Diane, how would you like an opportunity to grow and practice your confrontation skills?"

"I would hate it," she replied grinning. "I hate it that you said it that way."

Together we went into my office and did some role playing. She pretended that she was the volunteer, and I role modeled some possible scripts. Tentatively, but successfully, Diane was able to approach the volunteer with her concerns.

Fast-forward two years: Agnes arrives for the 3–11 shift. She is not just any nurse. This is Agnes the strong, Agnes the powerful. Agnes can bulldoze you with just a glance. Her words have the same effect as a typhoon. Every floor has an Agnes.

Upon hearing that she must float to another unit, Agnes voices her negativity for all to hear and storms off the floor, leaving an emotional trail of anger and guilt behind.

Diane chases her down and pulls her into the waiting area. She intends to give Agnes feedback about how those comments made everyone feel—and she does so with compassion, integrity, and grace. As a result, Agnes feels heard and understands the effect of her negative behavior.

There is nothing as rewarding as seeing your staff grow in skill, understanding, and compassion for others. The charge nurse retreat, shared mentoring of new staff, and role modeling of confrontation skills gave charge nurses the tools they needed to create a healthy culture. Slowly, they began to see how their presence, actions, and words could make a critical difference in their work environment.

Role modeling

Prior to each staff meeting, I meet with the charge nurses. Meetings are always an opportunity for staff or managers to bring up difficult or touchy issues—if there is an open system of communication. "A workplace is dysfunctional to the extent that unconscious forces are allowed to predominate in worker interactions, boss-worker relationships, or in leadership decisions" (Hart 1993). I was determined not to let these unconscious forces create a toxic environment on our unit.

One month, our staff education meeting focused on the importance of positive feedback in building a healthy community. I started by going around the room and complimenting each of the charge nurses on something very specific. Then we each wrote a thank you note to a staff member who went out of his or her way to do something that made the whole floor run more smoothly in the last week. These cards were truly appreciated by staff.

But it wasn't until the actual staff meeting that the charge nurses and staff finally realized the impact of their culture of stingy compliments.

I turned to a new resident nurse, who had just finished her three-month orientation, and asked, "Has anyone paid you a compliment in your three months here?" She was superb—confident, independent, caring, and very intelligent, so I didn't at all anticipate what happened next.

With tears streaming down her face, Julie shook her head and replied, "No."

There was not a person in that room whose heart did not go out to Julie or who, after seeing her pain, did not apologize and promise to themselves to be more generous with kind words. The key to decreasing horizontal hostility is to show its effect. **A manager's role is to bring our destructive practices from the darkness into the light.**

Fewer than half of the nurses in Aiken's five-country study (addressed in Chapter 1) reported that management acknowledged and valued their contributions (Aiken 2001). Managers have had a tendency to comment on "what is being done wrong, rather than what is being done right" (Thomas 2003). "Favorable recognition was a significant predictor of job satisfaction in Blegen's meta-analysis of 48 studies involving more than 15,000 nurses" (Thomas 2003). Clearly, compliments and recognition increase nurses' feelings of worth and value, thereby raising their self-esteem.

Performance evaluations

It is not easy to change a culture. At times, it feels like I'm swimming against a strong current. When depressed, I sing, "Me and Me Against the World" or "Alone Again, Naturally" in the elevator. I can get pretty maudlin and discouraged trying to decrease hostility and build a healthy work environment. Sometimes, I run to my office and tap out a quick e-mail to Oprah, which makes me feel better. The moments that rejuvenate me, however, are the precious conversations I have with staff—in just one meaningful interaction with a staff member, I realize again that we are *all* caught in this undertow of emotions. Every day, the pressures of our job and horizontal hostility take our profession way off course.

I once asked a peer how she was coping with the increased workload, hoping to hear some solutions I could apply myself. "I ask staff to fill out their own performance evaluations, and then I just sign them. I don't have time to meet with them," she said. I was really concerned. Had the demands of our jobs gotten to the point that we could not have just one conversation a year with our staff?

Performance evaluations are a golden opportunity to connect with a staff member on a more meaningful and deeper level than we ever could in a conversation on the floor. If this connection is compassionate, they in turn bring that compassion and understanding to the unit. The quality of relationship that we develop and demonstrate with staff becomes the standard for the unit and decreases horizontal hostility, one nurse at a time.

A silent witness is an accomplice

Audrey is the sweetest person on our floor. She is consistently pleasant, is clinically competent, and is a team player who steps up to the role of relief charge when needed. What more could I possibly say?

A section of our performance evaluations is marked "goals." I asked Audrey what she thought of the goal I had written on her performance evaluation: "Do not stand by and say nothing while staff are gossiping. Either walk away or point out that it is gossip and then walk away." She paused and responded thoughtfully, "That would stretch me . . . a lot."

Aware of the fact that Audrey herself would never gossip, I asked that she take a stand. Rather than be a silent witness to the drama, I asked that she deal with negative comments made about others in an assertive manner. Then came her questions.

"How do you do that? What do you say?" she asked.

We role played some scenes she had witnessed and discussed some scripts. The essence of the conversation was that it would take a lot of courage for her to actually say something or walk away. But the effects of "just standing by" and listening to negative comments were not benign. I focused on what emotions listening to people being criticized brought up for her. Then I asked how she would feel if she had walked away or told others how badly the negative gossip affected her. The feeling of self-respect that came with speaking her truth won by a long shot.

In summary, there are numerous ways to enhance communication and build a solid communication network on the unit. Leadership skills in charge nurses and key players are crucial and can be developed by

- holding charge nurse retreats
- encouraging a hierarchy of voice
- creating individual action plans
- creating a safe atmosphere
- role modeling crucial conversations
- empowering managers as leaders
- recognizing each other (i.e., using the power of a compliment)
- increasing knowledge and awareness about others' scope of responsibility
- instilling a new belief system

Response

"[It is] nurses themselves, who in their everyday work and interpersonal interactions, act as insidious gatekeepers to an iniquitous status quo."

—*Farrell (2001)*

A twofold approach

"Status quo" is an energetic equilibrium. If you take away something (hostility), you need to replace it with something else (healthy work practices). Executed exclusively, either of these actions will fail. Therefore, the most effective plan to eliminate horizontal hostility contains two critical actions. At the same time, leaders must

- **decrease** negativity, gossip, and a culture of blame by maintaining zero tolerance for any communication that is unhealthy, disrespectful, or spoken to people other than the person(s) directly involved

- **increase** a climate of safety and healthy communication by role modeling and using as many opportunities as possible to teach interpersonal and confrontation skills

Nurses decide what behavior is acceptable or unacceptable by how leaders respond to it. Our response is the only way to create new norms. Clearly, the manager would intervene if there was an angry, emotional, derogatory outburst, but what about the covert behaviors?

"In a healthy organization, every effort should be made to see to it that unconscious actions or motivations are brought out into the open" (Hart 1993). Some managers would think it trivial to follow up on a nurse who rolled her eyes when she found out whom she was working with that day. But it has been my experience that this eye rolling didn't just occur on the particular day you witnessed the behavior. I will bet that it happens every day with the same nurses, and that it affects the work climate by making everyone uncomfortable.

Check it out. To uncover covert behaviors, be vigilant. Arrange a time to meet with employees, and create a safe setting so that staff can tell you how they feel, which drives how they behave. Following up on overt and covert hostility in a timely manner is vital (even though some may argue that it is futile). Healing one relationship at a time, by taking consistent action, is the only way to communicate which behaviors are acceptable and which are unacceptable. Your consistent response is the strongest message you can possibly send, so follow up on *every* incident of hostility.

Typhoon Mary

She is stocky, strong willed, opinionated, judgmental, and a damn good nurse. Yesterday, she came in early for her shift, and the call lights were going off. Very irritated, Mary turned to the staff at the main station and loudly asked, "Isn't anyone going to get those call lights?! Doesn't anyone hear them but me?!"

No one moved. Now, even more annoyed, she charged into my office ranting about the "lazy" day shift. I asked her to come back after report.

As soon as the coast was clear, the charge nurse came in my office. "I heard her," she said flatly, "but I ignored her. I just can't stand that incriminating tone of voice. I know we should've heard the lights. It's been an insane day, and everyone just sat down to chart. It's just the way she says it that turns me off."

In my meeting with Mary, it took several minutes for her to admit that no one had listened to her. Emphatically, she said that she got along with everyone—"except for the two new orientees you hired who weren't any good." Mary spoke of how she expected a certain standard of care and was not, under any circumstances, going to settle for less. Was she the only one who cared around here?

I supported her values and desire to provide the best quality care, but I disagreed with her that she got along with everyone. Although that was Mary's perception, it was far from the truth. Weary of her tirades, staff just tuned her out. Tactfully, gently, I pointed that out.

"You are such a powerful woman, Mary. Your presence has so much energy. My goal is that when you speak to people, you really stop and hear what you are saying. I want staff to know of your good intentions and respect your knowledge. I want everyone to look to you to share your great skill. How would that feel?"

Some moments you never forget. I let the feeling of being heard, respected, and acknowledged settle over and absorb into her. Like a mirror, I held up a new image—one that she liked very much. And so we began our work. You would not recognize her today.

How do you deal with loud, strong, opinionated staff? You affirm how powerful they are, harness their energy and passion, and reframe their self-images so that all can appreciate them. Consider the analogy of a sailboat: The bigger the sail, the louder the sound it makes when there is no wind. In the past, addressing strong personalities has consisted mainly of taking the wind out of their sails, but it is far more effective to teach strong-willed staff how to *catch the wind.*

Response time is critical

Last year, two children died in foster care in the state of Washington. The governor's response included a new law: Events must be reported within 24 hours and acted upon within 72 hours. I use the same guidelines for dealing with horizontal hostility.

Staff have a tendency to minimize and dismiss hostile behavior if a week or so goes by and you are still investigating. You will hear, "Oh, don't worry about it," "It's okay, really," "I'm over it," "No big deal," etc. There is a clear window of opportunity during which the hostile behavior meant something to staff. The best time to intervene is when emotions are running strong. In addition, the majority of nurses tell a coworker when the hostile behavior occurs, so remember to address the whole unit or group rather than just the individuals involved (Farrell 2005).

Persistence and consistency is mandatory

It takes years of consistent intervening and mentoring to change any ingrained behavior. At no time can a leader "let that one go." A wise friend once told me that changing the practices or behaviors of a culture is like using the "Dead Man's Throttle" of a train: "You have to keep your hand on the throttle at all times or the train will stop." All of the above interventions, used consistently over a period of two years, *began* to decrease hostility and build a healthy work environment at our facility.

Empowering staff

When the pride and esteem of a few nurses soars, it raises the esteem of the entire group. I encouraged and helped staff to apply to speak at their national conference. The nurses' knowledge and expertise was validated and their esteem soared when their application was accepted. They were honored and excited to be presenting, and when an opportunity for staff to speak at an all-day high school conference arose, they eagerly accepted. The nurses then resurrected their annual regional conference, which had not happened in years. Staff nurses came forward and asked if they could do it again—and put the entire conference together by themselves! A sense of group pride emerged as these events raised the esteem of the unit.

Summary

Plan of care to eliminate horizontal hostility

1. Adopt a twofold approach
   a. Decrease hostility; adopt a zero-tolerance policy
   b. Increase skills and knowledge around a healthy workplace
2. Be aware of the signs and symptoms of horizontal hostility
3. Verbalize awareness of the problem to all staff—never ignore hostile behaviors
4. Establish a supportive and open communication network
   a. Offer opportunities for socialization
5. Set clear expectations—hold the vision, paint the picture
6. Demonstrate the effect—hold crucial conversations at every opportunity

7. Education

    a. Hold inservices on assertiveness training, confrontation, and crucial–conversation skills

    b. Replace the old belief system with a new one

    c. Create a new unit philosophy

    d. Encourage compliments

8. Increase the communication and conflict management skills of leaders

    a. Mentor key staff or charge nurses

    b. Establish a strong, open communication network

9. Respond in a timely and consistent manner

Recommended reading

Changing nurses' dis-empowering relationship patterns. *Journal of Advanced Nursing.*

    By Isolde Daiski

Bibliography

Aiken, L. et al. 2001. Nurses' reports on hospital care in five countries. *Health Affairs* 20(3): 43–53.

Blegen, M. 1993. Nurses' job satisfaction: a meta-analysis of related variables. *Nursing Research* 42(1): 36–41.

DeMarco, R., S. Roberts, and G. Chandler. 2005. The use of a writing group to enhance voice and connection among staff nurses. *Journal for Nurses in Staff Development* 21(3): 85–90.

Farrell, G. 2001. From tall poppies to squashed weeds: Why don't nurses pull together more? *Journal of Advanced Nursing* 35(1): 26–33.

Farrell, G. 2005. Violence in the Workplace Conference. Tualatin, Oregon. Sponsored by the Oregon Chapter of the American Psychiatric Nurses Association.

Hart, A. 1993. *The Crazy-Making Workplace*. Ann Arbor, MI: Servant Publications.

Namie, G., and R. Namie. 2000. *The Bully at Work: What You Can Do to Stop the Hurt and Reclaim Your Dignity on the Job*. Naperville, IL: Sourcebooks, Inc.

Scholtes, P. 1988. *The Team Handbook*. Madison, WI: Joiner Associates, Inc.

Thomas, S. 2003. 'Horizontal Hostility': Nurses against themselves: how to resolve this threat to retention. *Journal of Advanced Nursing* 103(10).

Wheatley, M. 2002. *Turning to One Another: Simple Conversations to Restore Hope to the Future*. San Francisco, CA: Berrett-Koehler Publishers.

Organizational opportunities

"It's not about what the organization does—it's what they don't do."
—Namie and Namie, The Bully at Work

Years ago, at a National League of Nursing meeting, Loretta Nowakowski, former director for Health Education for the Public at Georgetown University School of Nursing in Washington, DC, proposed that disease could be best understood by looking at hurricanes. She noted that, like a serious illness, hurricanes occurred only when many factors (variables) were present within relatively narrow parameters and that an appropriate intervention could alter the severity or course of a disease or hurricane. This discovery was encouraging to Nowakowski—it meant that an intervention, made at any point, could alter the final outcome.

And so it is with horizontal hostility. Our history, gender, education and work practices, interpersonal relationships, communication skills, organizational structure, etc., all contribute to producing horizontal hostility. The "hurricane" of horizontal hostility cannot manifest without these predisposing factors, so to intervene anywhere in this vast array can change the outcome from hostile to healthy.

The good news is that no matter what our current role—whether CNO, staff nurse, director, educator, or manager—we can implement interventions that will decrease hostility. Multiple opportunities are available at various levels.

Framework for leading organizational change to eliminate hostility

"Power is the ability to mobilize resources and get things done."

—*Kanter (1979)*

Enacting a twofold method (i.e., increasing a healthy environment while *simultaneously* decreasing hostility) is the most essential approach that managers can take to enact change at the organizational level.

To increase a healthy culture, managers must
- firmly establish senior leadership team commitment
- create infrastructures to support managers and staff
- provide a constructive feedback system for accountability and performance
- provide leadership training and confrontation skills training for managers
- provide assertiveness training and crucial-conversation training for staff
- monitor the organizational climate
- increase social capital—build a strong informal network

To decrease hostility, managers must
- adopt a zero-tolerance policy for horizontal hostility
- provide leadership training for managers
- educate staff about the effects of hostility

- create a system for reporting and monitoring
- participate with other hospitals to pass state legislation

Increase a healthy culture

Garner commitment from senior leadership

Eliminating horizontal hostility at an organizational level begins with a team commitment from senior leadership. Although this may seem obvious, the concept must be restated to prevent the "obvious" from being overlooked.

Commitment should stem from an awareness and understanding of the detrimental effects of hostility to morale and teamwork. Senior leaders also must realize that one of the greatest weaknesses of being at "the top of the food chain" is that you don't necessarily receive accurate, honest information. By its nature, a hierarchical "top-down" infrastructure discourages the upward flow of information.

"After hearing that I had received a job offer from another hospital, several physicians called the CEO to complain, who then called me down to his office. Since I already had a job offer, I had nothing to lose by telling the truth.

Boldly, I said, 'I hate to tell you, but you are naked. It's like the story "The Emperor's New Clothes" . . . you don't have anything on but you think you do. At other hospitals where I interviewed, I would have half the staff and double the support, yet you keep saying that this is the best place to work. It's not.' "

Applying theory to practice

As discussed earlier, the oppression theory is extremely helpful in understanding the basic dynamics of hostility and the behavioral characteristics of oppressed groups. It gives us a starting point and a framework from which to understand hostility. Now we need to view the larger picture: Hostility is not limited to staff nurses, but rather it is an "abusive and harmful activity perpetuated within organizations" (Hutchinson et al. 2006). At the heart of the matter is a diffuse and invisible force as strong as gravity: power. The question then becomes how is power given or withheld in our daily work practices?

Example: A new nurse meets with her manager and asks, "How long is my orientation?" The manager responds, "Three months." Contrast this to the manager who responds by saying, "As long as you need. Why don't you let me know when you feel ready and safe and we'll meet." Power pervades organizations in extremely subtle ways.

Infrastructure

Like new nurses, senior nurses ache for recognition in their daily work, the opportunity to tell their story, meaningful relationships with a mentor, and a set of skills that will enable them to work in a healthy environment. Yet the current infrastructure in hospitals is not set up to provide this level of support to staff. Nurses have no time for reflective practice, barely see their managers, and don't feel that their opinions matter. Their work is invisible to society, to the patient, and even to their own managers.

This situation is a Petri dish for horizontal hostility. Rosabeth Kanter's theory states that social structure is critical: "Situational conditions can constrain optimal job performance and, therefore, lower organizational productivity" (Kanter 1979). For example, a recent study of staff nurse empowerment showed that staff nurses with a chief nurse executive in a line structure felt significantly more empowered in their access to resources. (Matthews et al. 2006). Clearly, adopting an infrastructure that supports senior nurses would benefit both the individual nurse and the organization in creating a healthy work environment.

With our current infrastructure, a manager has a very slim chance of being successful in the leadership role. Kanter describes power as "the ability to get things done." Managers, however, lack the time and resources necessary to motivate and lead groups of people. Essentially, they lack power. Administrative and clerical tasks such as writing schedules, fulfilling competencies, preparing evaluations, updating standards, and instituting new procedures take up such a huge amount of time that there is no time for bonding and mentoring.

One recognized cost-reduction strategy of the 1990s restructuring was to expand a manager's scope of practice—especially in patient care areas. Span of control (i.e., the number of staff reporting to a manager, and not the number of FTEs) influences patient and staff outcomes. There is a demonstrated relationship between the number of staff reporting to a manager and patient satisfaction: The higher the number of nurses reporting, the lower the patient satisfaction rate. In an empirical study performed at a large Midwest health system, researchers also found that there was a relationship between employee engagement and span of control (Cathcart et al. 2004): As workgroup size increased, employee engagement decreased. Most importantly, the positive effects of leadership have been shown to decrease as span of control increases (Doran et al. 2004).

We desperately need engagement in nursing. We need involvement, buy-in, and a sense of belonging in order to establish a foundation for our work practice and any semblance of solidarity. We need leaders who can articulate and sustain a common vision, call people on their behavior, and role model new communication and confrontation skills. Without a connection between staff and their managers, the virulence and prevalence of horizontal hostility will only increase.

But research shows that "it is not humanly possible to consistently provide positive leadership to a very large number of staff while at the same time ensuring the effective and efficient operation of a large unit on a daily basis" (Doran et al. 2004). Therefore, a large span of control does not support nursing leadership. What type of infrastructure could possibly foster the level of support needed for a manager to institute the interventions discussed in Chapter 6?

Infrastructure considerations

Any infrastructure that levels the playing field, empowers nurses by giving them voice, elevates the visibility and value of nursing, and eliminates hierarchy will significantly decrease oppression, thereby decreasing horizontal hostility. **It is the struggle for a finite amount of power that provides the momentum for horizontal hostility.** But if a strong leader holds up a common vision—a vision of a workplace where everyone's unique contributions are acknowledged and valued— then an infinite amount of power becomes available. Staff united in a common goal (to create a healthy work environment) tap into a vast resource of infinite power, which in turn empowers them.

Assess span of control

Employee satisfaction surveys contain a wealth of information about the climate on a unit and the supervisor's ability to engage staff. Using this information to assess leader effectiveness and span of control is crucial. Not only should low scores be noted and plans be made for improvement, but the scores for a unit must be compared year to year. If morale, intent to leave, and overall satisfaction scores are very low, resurvey staff within six months.

Shared governance

Shared governance is a decentralized structure in which 90% of the decisions are made at the point of service (Porter O'Grady 2005). Moving decision-making to the bedside decreases hierarchy and therefore oppression, which alters the power infrastructure. Shared governance empowers nurses at the bedside. Nurses realize that they make a difference, that they are heard, and that they can exercise control over their work practice.

The role of empowerment in creating autonomy and job satisfaction is well known. Research shows that higher levels of workplace empowerment are positively related to perceptions of autonomy, control, and collaboration (Almost et al. 2003). Shared governance empowers nurses, and higher levels of empowerment increase job satisfaction and promote a healthy environment.

Shared governance benefits individuals as much as it benefits the organization. "Research has shown that the most cost-effective models are those models where accountability is at the point of service. In decentralized decision-making models, clinical outcomes, patient care, patient satisfaction, and patient/clinical efficacy are more advanced" (Porter O'Grady 2005).

ANCC Magnet Recognition Program® status

Nurses in ANCC Magnet Recognition Program®-accredited hospitals experience higher levels of empowerment and job satisfaction because they have greater access to organizational infrastructures that support them. In a study comparing Magnet status and non-Magnet status hospitals, greater visibility of nurse leaders, better support for autonomous decision-making, and greater access to information, resources, and opportunities were the three main elements of job satisfaction and empowerment in Magnet-designated hospitals (Upenieks 2003).

These key elements decrease horizontal hostility. Greater visibility of nursing leaders allows closer monitoring of behaviors and practices on the unit and provides opportunities to interrupt old behavior patterns. Greater autonomy in decision-making gives voice to the nurse at the bedside and leads to empowerment and an increased sense of self-esteem. Access to information, resources, and opportunities gives nurses the tools they need to do their jobs. In addition, nurses who are taught about horizontal hostility learn to depersonalize the behavior.

There are many known characteristics of Magnet status hospitals that enhance nurse leader effectiveness (Upenieks 2003):

- Visible nurse executives who value nursing, and leaders who role model caring.

- An administrative team that listens and responds to staff needs, thus increasing value, worth, and self-esteem.

- Nurse executives who disseminate their power to directors/managers, thus decreasing hierarchy and power struggles.

- Empowered nurses at the bedside.

- Freedom, opportunity, and upward movement, which are the characteristics of an open system.

- Collaborative physician-nurse relationships, which level the playing field.

Manager empowerment

Education must be provided to managers so that they can lead the cultural change to eliminate hostility. According to Kanter, empowerment means having access to information and resources, and opportunities to learn and grow (Matthews et al. 2006). **Empowering staff to change a culture must begin with managers who themselves are convinced that they have the ability, means, and tools to change the situation—that is, who themselves are empowered.**

Managers have the opportunity to "paint a new picture"; to articulate and hold a vision of the unit where staff are valued, acknowledged, and respected; and to approach each individual staff member who is demonstrating hostile behaviors and say, "Here, try this on. What would a healthy work environment where you were truly appreciated and valued feel like?" That vision releases a tremendous amount of power and energy.

A constructive feedback system

Providing a constructive feedback system for accountability and performance is critical because hostile behaviors flourish in a culture of secrecy (i.e., a closed system). Peer feedback, such as 360-degree assessments of managers, can be very useful. Unfortunately, these reviews also may be used to perpetuate horizontal hostility and should be carefully monitored. Staff who feel threatened by a peer may use this opportunity for sabotage or backstabbing. Conversely, staff who carefully select who provides feedback for them (i.e., their friends/supporters) can get away with unacceptable behavior for years.

In general, however, peer feedback at all levels is illuminating. For example, the charge nurse assessment tool (Chapter 6) proved to be an important resource for our staff, allowing them to perceive themselves through the eyes of the people they supervised. Peer evaluations equalize the playing field and establish a professional atmosphere.

Leadership and confrontation skills

Holding staff accountable is a bedrock of quality care. What happens when leaders do not hold staff accountable? A cascade of predictable events unfolds:

A nurse reports an unacceptable behavior to his or her manager . . .

No action is taken . . .

The nurse feels helpless ("What difference does it make?") . . .

The behavior continues and the feeling of helplessness is reinforced . . .

It happens again and the nurse doesn't report it ("It makes no difference") . . .

The unacceptable behavior creates negativity that spreads insidiously . . .

Staff who were once just witnesses of the behavior become victims of it . . .

The behavior is copied by others who see no consequences . . .

No one bothers reporting any further incidents ("What difference does it make?") . . .

"Aggression breeds aggression" (Farrell 2005) in the workplace . . .

and horizontal hostility becomes the culture.

Everyone in a leadership position, from charge nurses to administration, must acquire the skill set necessary to confront others. These skills, typically lacking in our educational programs, must become integral to the curriculum.

Offering education in any of the following areas will help create a healthy environment:

- Assertiveness training for all staff
- Crucial conversations
- Reflective practice
- Physician-nurse education and networking
- Conflict management and confrontation skills

Assertiveness training and crucial conversations

"The void created by the failure to communicate is soon filled with poison, drivel, and misrepresentation."

—C. Northcote Parkinson (Patterson et al. 2002)

Classes designed to improve communication skills are mandatory to confront hostile behaviors. Nurses have demonstrated time and again that their communication skill set is inadequate and ineffective—they will tell everyone on the entire floor why they are angry except the person with whom they are angry. This practice is interpreted as a lack of respect and perpetuates more negative behaviors. Classes to prevent such behaviors should focus on crucial conversations, conflict management, confrontation skills, and assertiveness training.

Crucial conversations are discussions between two or more people in which the stakes are high, opinions vary, and emotions are running strong (Patterson et al.

2002)—the daily environment in most hospitals. Stakes are always high when a group must struggle for the resources they need to do their jobs (as is characteristic of an oppressed culture). Multiple opinions grow out of conflicting vested interests. When every department is struggling to stay under budget, a change in practice or a "process improvement" can result in another department having to assume increased costs. Not only does conflict ensue, but subtle task shifts often go unnoticed.

"We just deliver the food trays; we don't pick them up."

"I know the new food and drug interaction policy requires a pharmacist to counsel patients on the first dose, but I don't have the staff to meet that requirement."

Emotions are running strong in nursing because nurses
- do not have an outlet for frustration
- do not have an opportunity to process or reflect on their experiences
- are wounded by horizontal hostility
- lack a support system/solidarity
- have adapted to an increased pace of work

Because these crucial conversations are not happening, the work environment abounds in unexpressed negative emotions. Nurses avoid conversations that "take too much energy" or handle them poorly because they are too emotionally engaged (Patterson et al. 2002). The passive-aggressive communication style characteristic of nurses also contributes to this avoidance of the issue. Nursing desperately needs a skill set that instructs staff on how to recognize a crucial conversation and how to find the "shared pool of meaning."

When we as managers deal with conflict, the stakes are always high. There is a long history of staff feeling threatened and judged. As we develop our abilities to create a "safe" conversation zone, we role model a new skill set that encourages other nurses to do the same.

Assertiveness training and communication skills training have proven to be effective intervention tools in reducing hostile behavior in the operating room (Cook et al. 2001). This fact applies to other areas as well. Some researchers also advocate early interventions, counseling, and formal education programs to catch the behavior before it escalates (Anderson and Stamper 2001). This education includes providing examples of hostility during hospital orientation, as well as offering training on how to handle these incidents. Assertiveness training empowers staff and moves them out of the victim role.

Another opportunity to build a culture of healthy relationships is to encourage relationships between staff and physicians. Creating social and networking opportunities enables physicians and nurses to get to know each other beyond work roles. This personal connection levels the playing field and strengthens relationships. When physician department heads and unit managers work together on hospital initiatives, staff perceive a united front and common goal.

Organizational climate

Culture is crucial to an organization. Like the air we breathe, it can be either toxic and poisoning or fresh and invigorating. As nurses come onto a shift, just one biting comment muttered under someone's breath can set a negative tone for the next eight hours. The toxic climate that results is not healthy for patients or staff.

Organizational climate, which is established by leaders, is a direct result of our interpersonal relationships. Thus, assessing the quality of relationships will yield a great deal of information. Do you hear frequent complaints? Are compliments given? What is the level of communication and camaraderie at meetings?

To assess the organizational climate, the mental/emotional health of staff should be measured and improvement plans put in place as needed. After assessments are conducted and the results become available, follow up with any staff who have indicated a problem. This critical step indicates to staff that they are cared about and valued.

Areas that experience high turnover and absenteeism or have many physician complaints should set off a red flag. To prevent turnover and give leaders the information they need, exit interviews should be mandatory and performed at least two levels above the employee's current level.

Social capital

Social capital describes the very fabric of our connections with each other. Over the past two generations, social capital has dramatically decreased as Americans have steadily dropped out of organized community activities (Putnam 2000). The social capital in nursing also has decreased tremendously, especially over the last decade. The impact of increased acuity, technology, pharmacology, and patient-staff ratios, combined with a decreased length of stay, has significantly decreased social capital.

"Social capital turns out to have forceful, even quantifiable effects on many different aspects of our lives . . . Networks of community engagement foster sturdy norms of reciprocity. The positive consequence of social capital have been noted to be: mutual support, cooperation, trust, and institutional effectiveness" (Putnam 2000). Thus, it is clear that possessing a fair amount of social capital in nursing would decrease hostility and improve the work environment.

The decrease of involvement in community, in both the social and the nursing realms, has resulted in an increase in isolation and a decrease in opportunities to practice our social skills. The more "productive" we are, the less time we have to bond and network with each other. In our current way of doing business, if you are at a maximum point for productivity and efficiency, then social capital is minimally available. There is an inverse relationship between productivity/efficiency and social capital.

"They called me the floater," said Harry.

"What's that?" I asked.

"Well, on my breaks or during the shift, I would go to other departments and check out how they were doing. I would go to the ICU or the lab and visit. I would talk to people and, you know, check in. It was really nice. I knew everybody."

"When was the last time you did that?" I asked.

"Oh, about 15 years ago," he replied.

Social capital is a mandatory component of solidarity (Putnam 2000). There is tremendous power available in the informal network of relationships that supports any organization. Capitalizing on this power by creating social and networking opportunities will strengthen the fabric of any organization.

"[The doctor] couldn't have told you my name, despite the fact that I worked full-time on the floor for five years. Then one weekend it was slow, and he wasn't in a hurry as usual, so we started talking and found out that our kids were on the same soccer team. Not only does he know my name now, but he looks at me like I'm a person, not 'the nurse.' He's so much more receptive to my suggestions for patient care."

Decrease hostility

Zero tolerance for horizontal hostility

Obtaining honest and accurate information in an oppressive culture can be a challenge. How do you get it? By adopting a zero-tolerance rule for hostile behavior. Commitment to this policy will open the lines of communication, encourage the reporting of such events, and support the upward flow of information.

On our unit, the zero-tolerance policy for hostility came from our group of nursing assistants. After mandatory meetings designed to empower the assistants (two hours bimonthly for two years), the nursing assistants felt a strong sense of identity and solidarity. After a rather emotional week of gossip that could rival any soap opera, the nursing assistants decided that people talking behind each others' backs was completely unacceptable. They instituted a policy that if you had something to say, you needed to go to the person involved and speak to them in private. The nursing assistants wholeheartedly embraced this new policy, which was then adopted by all staff.

Staff began to realize that they could not possibly create a healing environment for patients because backstabbing and gossip made working as a team impossible. What motivated them was seeing and feeling the damage that hostility caused and realizing that they had the power to change the situation.

Why did this policy originate in the nursing assistant group rather than in staff meetings? Because the group was much smaller (12), which made it feasible to have mandatory meetings that focused on their particular issues, taught assertiveness skills, and encouraged them to develop solutions. This time together was something the other nurses clearly did not have, and this education empowered the nursing assistants.

For instance, at one of their meetings, the nursing assistants vented that they felt pulled in a million directions at once and were frustrated. When they were in the middle of bathing a patient, someone would ask them to do something else, and with a number of staff making requests, no one saw the stress of these multiple demands. So for our next class, we focused on communication skills. I taught the assistants some scripts they could use when frustrated like, "I can be there in five minutes" or "I'm in the middle of a bath, can someone else help?"

The *very first* time a nursing assistant used this script, there was a loud knock on my door. An angry nurse burst into my office saying, "What bull are you teaching these assistants that they can actually say 'no'?"

When this story was shared with the charge nurses, they began to better understand the oppression within our own workgroup.

Unit-based policies generated by staff are very effective, yet they must fall under the larger umbrella of a corporate/organizational policy in order to have Human Resources support. Also, make sure the policies are written in clear, simple language and are easy to understand. Because this is a complex subject that nurses do not wish to acknowledge, education must accompany implementation.

Education about policies must
- help staff understand horizontal hostility and its impact
- teach staff how to access the zero-tolerance policy, how to report hostility, and how to find out that the issue has been addressed
- clearly define unacceptable behaviors (give examples)
- ensure that the policy has exposure on all levels

In order to support zero tolerance for hostility, behavioral standards should be included in performance evaluations. If they are not, then there is no way for management to hold staff accountable for them.

At Orange Regional Medical Center in Middletown, NY, a Standards of Performance and Behavior policy was created for all employees (see Figure 7.1). According to Nursing Director Eva Edwards, these standards highlight basic manners for employees to follow. Prior to the policy's implementation, each employee met with his or her manager to discuss the standards and the organization's expectation of adhering to them. Those employees who refused to sign because they knew that they would not be able to live up to the standards were given guidance to help them reach the organization's expectations.

| **Figure 7.1** | **Commitment to coworkers** |

"It is much easier to build a good relationship than to struggle with a bad one."

- We will maintain a supportive attitude with peers, creating a positive team environment by recognizing our colleagues for performance that exceeds expectations. We will hold each other accountable for our behavior and performance, recognizing that the actions of one speak for the entire team.

- We recognize that each of us plays a vital role in this facility's operations and treat each other accordingly.

- Rudeness is never tolerated.

- There is no blaming, finger pointing, or undermining our fellow employees or those in other departments.

- We are on time for our shifts, for our meetings, and when returning from breaks.

- We treat each other as professionals with courtesy, honesty, and respect.

- We welcome and nurture newcomers.

- We recognize that many hands make light work and offer to help each other.

- We show appreciation and support to staff that come to our aid from other units and departments.

Figure 7.1   **Commitment to coworkers (cont.)**

- We do not call in sick unless we are sick.

- We recognize that we all have strengths and weaknesses and that it takes many diverse personalities to make a team.

- We respect cultural differences in one another.

- We praise each other in public and criticize in private.

- We do not gossip. We protect the privacy and feelings of our fellow employees.

- We profess that "There is no 'I' in 'TEAM.' "

- Our actions and attitudes make our fellow employees feel appreciated, included, and valued.

- Staff and leaders share ideas and openly communicate with each other.

- We respect each other's time and avoid urgent requests.

- We have fun and keep a sense of humor at work.

Source: Orange Regional Medical Center, Middletown, NY. Reprinted with permission.

Leadership training for managers

Adopting a zero-tolerance policy for staff will mean nothing if front-line leaders do not have the leadership skills necessary to hold staff accountable. Above all, managers must be able to articulate and sustain a clear vision. They need to motivate and empower staff to change a negative nursing environment into a healthy workplace. They must be leaders.

Many nurses and managers have become so acculturated that they do not even see the negative effects of hostile behaviors. The only way to demonstrate the impact is to demonstrate the effect—the hurt and the pain—of the behavior. However, managers/leaders who have visibility and presence on the unit and who have established an open communication network can do so by confronting staff and holding crucial conversations.

A system for reporting and monitoring

The very first stumbling block to reporting and monitoring is the "What difference does it make?" attitude that prevails in nursing. If staff had seen effective actions taken in the past, we wouldn't have this problem. The only way staff will report the overt and covert behaviors characteristic of hostility is if they see that their reporting stops the behavior. That's why mastering confrontation and conflict management skills is critical for managers.

Systems for reporting must be anonymous, safe, and easily available. An online reporting tool would work well. Our unit has a Web site with a "feedback" button that provides a secure link for staff members to send their concerns to me anonymously via e-mail, although this option is infrequently used now that face-to-face conversations have become the norm.

Note that managers themselves can also be a problem and that a hospital-wide reporting system is optimal. Be sure to monitor red flag areas of high staff turnover, absenteeism, or high-volume patient/physician/staff complaints.

State legislation

Hospitals must seize every opportunity to advocate for legislation at the local or state levels. Addressing the impact of horizontal hostility (especially during a severe nursing shortage) at state hospital board of association meetings will increase awareness and support.

How the system sets up the manager to fail

When resources are scarce, there is always a power struggle. Thus, in an attempt to stay financially viable, many organizational decisions have been made without sufficient consideration of their impact. To respond to this problem, initiate discussions with administration that address whether the system sets up the manager to fail and what can be done to rectify the problem.

Some commonly heard replies/complaints/suggestions from managers and directors may include the following:

- Span of control is not being addressed.

- Budgets are being created with little research and without the input of nursing support staff.

- Bad employees are being passed around.

- There is no Human Resources backup.

- Employees are promoted and then not given the tools and resources they need to succeed.

- There is a highly weighted focus on productivity/efficiency—and ignorance of the benefits of social bonding and networking.

- Upper management has "no idea what I actually do"/role ignorance. [Note: It should be mandatory that managers follow a nurse for an entire shift once a year, that a director follow a manager through her day, etc. "I was a manager once too, you know" doesn't cut it when you held that role twenty years ago. A clear and accurate picture of the challenges our subordinates face can only result in better support.]

- A constructive feedback system for accountability and performance is needed.

- Leadership training and confrontation skills training for managers is needed.

- Assertiveness training and crucial-conversation training for staff is needed.

- Monitor the organizational climate.

- Increase social capital—build a strong informal network.

Summary

Organizational strategies
1. Establish visible senior leadership team commitment
    a. Communicate the vision of a healthy work environment

2. Assess and address infrastructure needs

    a. Use the wealth of information available in employee satisfaction surveys

    b. Pursue a shared governance model/Magnet status

    c. Reexamine span of control

3. Institute policies

    a. Adopt a zero-tolerance policy for horizontal hostility

    b. Include behavioral standards in performance evaluations

    c. Require mandatory exit interviews with managers/leaders who are two levels above the employee's level

4. Provide education

    a. Create opportunities for reflective practice

    b. Provide classes on assertiveness training and crucial conversations

    c. Provide opportunities for physician-nurse education and networking

    d. Provide conflict management and confrontation skills classes for managers/leaders, as well as intense leadership training

5. Assess the cohesiveness and psychological safety of work groups

    a. Use nominal group technique or anonymous surveys to elicit information

    b. Create an anonymous reporting system, and monitor red-flag areas closely

6. Provide opportunities to increase social support network/bonding

    a. Make sure meetings include time to bond

    b. Make sure meetings are not simply a place to disseminate information

    c. Give managers and directors the opportunity to speak about their individual challenges and solutions

7. Participate with other hospitals to pass zero-tolerance legislation to protect nurses from hostility from peers, patients, and visitors

Recommended reading

Crucial Conversation: Tools for Talking When Stakes Are High
By Kerry Patterson et al.

Fierce Conversations: Achieving Success at Work & in Life, One Conversation at a Time
By Susan Scott

Leadership on the Line: Staying Alive through the Dangers of Leading
By Ronald A. Heifetz and Marty Linsky

Leadership and the New Science: Discovering Order in a Chaotic World
By Margaret J. Wheatley

Bibliography

Almost, J., H. Laschinger, and D. Tuer-Hodes. 2003. Workplace empowerment and Magnet hospital characteristics. *Journal of Nursing Administration* 33: 410–422.

Anderson, C., and M. Stamper. 2001. *Workplace violence.* RN 64(2): 71–74.

Cathcart, D. et al. 2004. Span of control matters. *Journal of Nursing Administration* 34(9): 395–399.

Cook, J. et al. 2001. Exploring the impact of physician verbal abuse on perioperative nurses. *AORN Journal* 74(3): 317–330.

Doran, D. et al. 2004. Impact of the manager's span of control on leadership and performance. Canadian Health Services Research Foundation. *www.chsrf.ca.*

Farrell, G. 2005. Violence in the Workplace Conference. Tualatin, Oregon. Sponsored by the Oregon Chapter of the American Psychiatric Nurses Association. Hutchinson, M. et al. 2006. Workplace bullying in nursing: Towards a more critical organisational perspective. *Nursing Inquiry* 13(2): 118-126.

Kanter, R. 1979. Power failure in management circuits. *Harvard Business Review* 57(4): 65–75.

Matthews, S. et al. 2006. Staff nurse empowerment in line and staff organizational structures for chief nurse executives. *Journal of Nursing Administration* (36)11.

Namie, G., and R. Namie, 2000. *The Bully at Work: What You Can Do to Stop the Hurt and Reclaim Your Dignity on the Job.* Naperville, IL: Sourcebooks, Inc.

Patterson, K. et al. 2002. Crucial Conversation: Tools for Talking When Stakes are High. New York: McGraw-Hill Trade.

Porter O'Grady, T. 2005. *Shared Governance: How to Create and Sustain a Culture of Nurse Empowerment.* Audioconference. HCPro, Inc.

Sapolsky, R. 1998. *Why Zebras Don't Get Ulcers: An Updated Guide to Stress, Stress-related Diseases and Coping.* New York: Freeman & Company.

Upenieks, V. 2003. The interrelationship of organizational characteristics of Magnet hospitals, nursing leadership and nursing job satisfaction. *Health Care Manager* 22(2): 83–97.

Individual response

"The future doesn't take form irrationally, even though it feels that way. The future comes from where we are now. It materializes from the actions, values, and beliefs we're practicing now. We're creating the future every day, by what we choose to do. If we want a different future, we have to take responsibility for what we are doing in the present."

—Wheatley (2002)

Starting with ourselves

After giving a speech at a small community hospital, I invited the audience to contact me with their stories of horizontal hostility. Immediately after I finished, five nurses came up to the front of the room to share their own experiences. Four of them were brand-new nurses. Concerned, I looked for the right moment to share this important information with the director.

"Did you notice the new grads coming up to the front of the room offering examples of horizontal hostility? They seemed pretty anxious to tell their stories."

"Did you see all the happy faces leaving the room?" she said, completely ignoring my remark.

"And yesterday was the same way," she continued. "It's so good to see the smiles on the nurses faces as they leave the retreat."

A few weeks later, I had lunch with a colleague of the director and told her what had happened.

"She's just overworked," the colleague replied. "There's a new computer project. She probably works 70 hours a week now. She just couldn't hear you," she said plainly.

And then she added, "She can't hear me either."

Before we begin illuminating the behavior of others, we must first illuminate our own. Regardless of our position, from educator to CNO to staff nurse, we must take a minute to assess the role we play in ending or perpetuating horizontal hostility in the workplace.

Research shows that staff nurses do not feel that telling a manager about hostility is an effective solution. After experiencing verbal abuse, 78% talk to a friend and 32% talk to a manager—but 10% of that 32% say that talking to a manager is of no help (Farrell 2005).

The insidious nature of horizontal hostility is the greatest problem. To bring hostility to light, we must show its effect. By doing so, the healing process can begin and genuine relationships can begin to take root. And as these meaningful relationships grow, not only will horizontal hostility decrease, but the solidarity we so desperately need in nursing will emerge.

Just as staff nurses have internalized overt and covert behaviors as normal, we as leaders have internalized practices that unconsciously perpetuate oppression.

"I was exasperated. In tears, I turned the corner and accidentally bumped into the Vice President of Human Resources. 'What's the matter?' she asked.

I didn't know where to start. 'We've had a 35% turnover in our manager group in less than a year. How high does that number have to be before you notice . . . before somebody cares? 50%? 100%?' "

"I told my director about the backstabbing and gossip. She was useless—turned it right back on me. Her only response was, 'Now why do you think someone would be so mean to you?' "

Due to the pressures outlined in Section I—including the power struggle that results from a scarcity of resources—nursing administration functions as a closed system, and closed systems are by nature dysfunctional.

Experienced nurses are very familiar with the story of the bucket of crabs. A man was walking by and saw a crab starting to crawl up and out of the bucket. Quickly, he told the kids, "You better put a lid on those crabs or they'll get out." But the kids responded, "Mister, everyone knows you don't need a lid on a bucket of crabs because every time one tries to escape, the other crabs pull it back down."

Like a bucket of crabs, any group of oppressed people will use degrading and dehumanizing overt and covert tactics to ensure that *all* members of the group are oppressed. There seems to be an unwritten rule that says, "If I have no power and am stuck in this mess, then everyone else should be too."

Transitioning from a closed system to an open system

One common observation from outsiders is the "above and beyond" amount of energy that nursing administrators typically pour into their work. Going far beyond the call of duty—often to the point of exhaustion—is characteristic of a closed system.

Other characteristics of a closed system include

- little professional or social contact with similar groups
- treating outsider and individual opinions with suspicion
- worker dysfunction, passed on from generation to generation
- an expectation that one must surrender one's personal and family life out of loyalty
- increased dependence on the job for social support (Hart 1993)
- fear of saying what one really thinks
- little to no social interaction
- all conversations at breaks or meal times dominated by work issues

Creating an open system would benefit administrators, nurse managers, educators, and staff alike, but it requires that we redefine our boundaries. Characteristics of an open system include

- mandatory "time-outs" at meetings for open forum, networking, or out-of-the-box thinking

- the sharing of struggles (e.g., brainstorming for solutions together, taking the time to share problems, and taking pride in the solutions)

- reasonable work hours

- time *and support* to participate in professional groups

- reasonable scope of practice

- the freedom, ability, and safety to say no and have it be heard

- mutual respect and admiration (i.e., zero cliques and zero gossip)

- leaders who report being energized from being in one another's presence

As Marie said, "We need each other." Nursing is difficult work. Building a new culture starts with rebuilding our relationships—one at a time. At this very moment, each of us knows the name of the person who *"doesn't respect me/doesn't like me/won't sit next to me/is putting me down."* And we know who we feel the same way about. Any hesitance to hold the crucial conversations necessary to heal these relationships must be immediately addressed, whether the relationships are with superiors, peers, or subordinates.

We can never expect staff to "go there" if we don't show them the way. It is not possible for solidarity and substantial culture changes to arise from the masses of nurses alone. They are completely focused on the daily struggles of the unit and are totally enmeshed in the nursing culture we are trying to illuminate.

Change simply will not happen unless nursing leadership takes on the challenge and the responsibility of making it happen. In the end, the nursing revolution we so desperately need in order to eliminate horizontal hostility will come from the deep and profound respect, compassion, and admiration we have for each other as nurses.

Bibliography

Farrell, G. 2005. Unpublished "SWAN" study presented at the "Violence in the Workplace" conference. Tualatin, OR. Sponsored by the Oregon Chapter of the American Psychiatric Nurses Association.

Hart, A. 1993. *The Crazy-Making Workplace*. Ann Arbor, MI: Servant Publications.

Wheatley, M. 2002. *Turning to One Another: Simple Conversations to Restore Hope to the Future*. San Francisco: Berrett-Koehler Publishers.

Epilogue

The etymology of a word often provides us with insight that is not always obvious in the simple definition.

In the end, it comes down to respect. According to the American Heritage® Dictionary, the etymology of the word "respect" is "from Middle English, *regard*, from Old French, from Latin *respectus*, from past participle of *respicere: to look back at, regard, consider.*"

Now, I want to go back to the hospital and find Skye. I have something to say . . .

In a nutshell, *we are not looking*. If we could take the time to be with and listen to each other, horizontal hostility could not exist. If we looked with compassion and intention into each other's eyes, we would see the two things we so desperately need to heal: *each other's pain and our own reflection.* There is so much strength and power available in that look, for in it we see our common humanity. As the author Eudora Welty so eloquently said of her work,

> "My continuing passion is to part a curtain,
> that invisible shadow that falls between people,
> the veil of indifference to each other's presence,
> each other's wonder, each other's human plight."

Nursing education instructional guide

Ending Nurse-to-Nurse Hostility:
Why Nurses Eat Their Young and Each Other

Target audience:

Nurse managers, staff nurses, and new resident/student nurses

Statement of need:

This book provides an educational guide for nurse managers to help them understand what horizontal hostility is, why it occurs and prevails in nursing, and how the situation can be remedied. By coupling anecdotal evidence and scenarios with tangible advice for nurses, the book offers field-tested, how-to advice for tackling horizontal hostility and teaches nurses how to put an end to it in their facilities and improve nursing culture. Strategies for recognizing and combating nurse-to-nurse hostility are discussed, as well as prevention methods.

Educational objectives:

Upon completion of this activity, participants should be able to

- Define horizontal hostility
- List two overt examples of horizontal hostility from the work setting
- List two covert examples of horizontal hostility from the work setting
- Discuss the impact that horizontal hostility has on 1) the individual and 2) the organization
- Explain the ways in which the current system is designed to support the invisibility of nurses
- List two populations at risk for experiencing horizontal hostility
- State four of the most frequent forms of lateral violence
- Explain why horizontal hostility is so virulent
- Identify two intrinsic forces that play a role in horizontal hostility
- Identify two extrinsic forces that play a role in horizontal hostility
- Explain how the organizational structure enables oppression
- Select two factors that contribute to nurses' stress from the context of our world
- List two impediments to a healthy student or resident nurse experience
- Describe six steps that can be taken to create a healthy environment for student nurses
- Name two signs of which managers should be aware that may indicate that horizontal hostility is taking place
- Explain what is meant by a "twofold approach" to eliminating horizontal hostility
- Select one way in which nurse managers can empower staff
- Identify two strategies to nurture a healthy culture within the organization
- Identify two strategies to decrease hostility within the organization
- Identify two practices or behaviors characteristic of a closed system

Author

Kathleen Bartholomew, RN, MN

Accreditation/designation statement:

This educational activity for four contact hours is provided by HCPro, Inc. HCPro is accredited as a provider of continuing nursing education by the American Nurses Credentialing Center's Commission on Accreditation.

Disclosure statements

Kathleen Bartholomew has declared that she has no commercial/financial vested interest in this activity.

Instructions for obtaining your nursing contact hours

In order to be eligible to receive your nursing contact hour(s) for this activity, you are required to do the following:

1. Read the book
2. Complete the exam
3. Complete the evaluation
4. Provide your contact information in the space provided on the exam and evaluation
5. Submit the exam and evaluation to HCPro, Inc.

Please provide all of the information requested above and mail or fax your completed exam, program evaluation, and contact information to

HCPro, Inc.
Attention: Kerry Betsold, Continuing Education Manager
200 Hoods Lane
P.O. Box 1168
Marblehead, MA 01945
Fax: 781/639-0179

If you have any questions, please contact our customer service department at 877/727-1728.

Nursing education exam

Name: _____

Title: _____

Facility name: _____

Address: _____

Address: _____

City: _____ State: _____ ZIP: _____

Phone number: _____ Fax number: _____

E-mail: _____

Nursing license number: _____

(ANCC requires a unique identifier for each learner)

1. **What is horizontal hostility, as defined by Farrell?**
   a. Nurses being mean to one another
   b. Infighting between two groups on the same professional level
   c. A consistent pattern of behavior designed to control, diminish, or devalue another
   d. Physical assault against a coworker

2. **Name-calling, gossip, and bickering are three examples of what type of hostility?**
   a. Overt
   b. Covert
   c. Severe
   d. Illegal

3. **Which of the following actions is an example of covert hostility?**
   a. Shouting
   b. Criticism
   c. Pushing
   d. Isolation

4. **Staff who have been bullied rate higher in what area?**
   a. Job performance
   b. Depression
   c. Emotional sensitivity
   d. Intelligence

5. **Daily failure to acknowledge nurses' contributions supports the _____ of nurses.**
   a. visibility
   b. education
   c. invisibility
   d. identity

6. **According to the text, new hires, transfers from other departments, and new resident nurses are all at high risk for experiencing horizontal hostility. Why?**

    a. They are not prepared to stand up for themselves.

    b. They do not understand the culture.

    c. They are abrasive.

    d. They are entering a powerless group.

7. **According to Figure 2.1, what is the most frequent form of lateral violence in nursing practice?**

    a. Shoving

    b. Backstabbing

    c. Nonverbal innuendo

    d. Sabotage

8. **Ineffective supervisor intervention contributes to the virulent nature of horizontal hostility. What is one of the reasons identified in the text for the manager's lack of response?**

    a. Poor conflict management skills

    b. Pressure from upper management to ignore the problem

    c. Sabotage

    d. Company policy

9. **What precipitates the emotional state of anger?**

    a. Jubilation

    b. Unfair or disrespectful treatment and/or a lack of reciprocity in relationships

    c. Divorce from a spouse

    d. Support from coworkers

10. According to the text, task and time imperatives lead nurses to see patients as _____.

    a. annoyances   c. relief from paperwork

    b. tasks   d. people

11. The ladder of hierarchy enables oppression in the organization. Where are nurses situated on the ladder?

    a. At the top   c. At the bottom

    b. In the middle   d. On another ladder

12. How has the national decrease in group membership contributed to nurses' stress?

    a. It has made them more isolated.

    b. It has made their children more independent.

    c. It has given them more free time.

    d. It has caused more medical problems.

13. Lacking an understanding of the pace of the floor, new nurses have the perception that they are "in the way." According to the text, this often leads to what?

    a. Patient satisfaction

    b. Feelings of rejection and a lack of bonding

    c. Nervous breakdowns

    d. Fatigue

14. In revising the curriculum (Step 5 of creating a healthy environment), what skills should be taught and practiced?

a. Time-management skills

b. Resolution skills

c. High-level communication and assertiveness skills

d. Finance and planning skills

15. What is one indication that horizontal hostility may be taking place?

a. Increased productivity

b. High retention rates

c. High turnover rates

d. High patient satisfaction

16. The twofold approach states that leaders must decrease negativity, gossip, and a culture of blame while simultaneously doing what?

a. Sending out assessments

b. Developing retention programs

c. Honoring preceptors

d. Increasing a climate of safety and healthy communication

17. Speaking engagements and presentations empower staff by

a. helping them earn money

b. validating their knowledge and raising self-esteem

c. getting them away from the unit/facility

d. making them more popular with their colleagues

18. **Putting infrastructures in place to support managers and staff is one way to increase a healthy culture. One infrastructure consideration indicated in the text that may empower nurses is**

    a. shared governance

    b. a larger facility

    c. an increase in the number of charge nurses

    d. taking the decision-making power out of nurses' hands

19. **Having a system in place for reporting and monitoring hostile behavior is one way to decrease hostility. What tool did the author use at her facility for reporting such incidents?**

    a. A form that could be handed in to the manager

    b. An online reporting tool that allows staff to remain anonymous

    c. A telephone hotline

    d. Face-to-face conversations with the perpetrator

20. **Little professional or social contact with similar groups and worker dysfunction are two examples of**

    a. a hostile system   c. an open system

    b. a healthy system   d. a closed system

Nursing education evaluation

Name: _____

Title: _____

Facility name: _____

Address: _____

Address: _____

City: _____ State: _____ ZIP: _____

Phone number: _____ Fax number: _____

E-mail: _____

Nursing license number: _____
(ANCC requires a unique identifier for each learner)

1. This activity met the following learning objectives:

Defined horizontal hostility

Strongly disagree 1   2   3   4   5   Strongly agree

Listed two overt examples of horizontal hostility from the work setting

Strongly disagree 1   2   3   4   5   Strongly agree

Listed two covert examples of horizontal hostility from the work setting

Strongly disagree 1   2   3   4   5   Strongly agree

Discussed the impact that horizontal hostility has on 1) the individual and 2) the organization

Strongly disagree 1   2   3   4   5   Strongly agree

Explained the ways in which the current system is designed to support the invisibility of nurses

Strongly disagree 1   2   3   4   5   Strongly agree

Listed two populations at risk for experiencing horizontal hostility

Strongly disagree 1   2   3   4   5   Strongly agree

Stated four of the most frequent forms of lateral violence

Strongly disagree 1   2   3   4   5   Strongly agree

Explained why horizontal hostility is so virulent

Strongly disagree 1   2   3   4   5   Strongly agree

Identified two intrinsic forces that play a role in horizontal hostility

Strongly disagree 1   2   3   4   5   Strongly agree

Identified two extrinsic forces that play a role in horizontal hostility

Strongly disagree 1   2   3   4   5   Strongly agree

Explained how the organizational structure enables oppression

Strongly disagree 1   2   3   4   5   Strongly agree

Selected two factors that contribute to nurses' stress from the context of our world

Strongly disagree 1   2   3   4   5   Strongly agree

Listed two impediments to a healthy student or resident nurse experience

Strongly disagree 1   2   3   4   5   Strongly agree

Described six steps that can be taken to create a healthy environment for student nurses
Strongly disagree 1   2   3   4   5   Strongly agree

Named two signs of which managers should be aware that may indicate that horizontal hostility is taking place
Strongly disagree 1   2   3   4   5   Strongly agree

Explained what is meant by a "twofold approach" to eliminating horizontal hostility
Strongly disagree 1   2   3   4   5   Strongly agree

Selected one way in which nurse managers can empower staff
Strongly disagree 1   2   3   4   5   Strongly agree

Identified two strategies to nurture a healthy culture within your organization
Strongly disagree 1   2   3   4   5   Strongly agree

Identified two strategies to decrease hostility within your organization
Strongly disagree 1   2   3   4   5   Strongly agree

Identified two practices or behaviors characteristic of a closed system
Strongly disagree 1   2   3   4   5   Strongly agree

2. Objectives were related to the overall purpose/goal of the activity.
Strongly disagree   1   2   3   4   5   Strongly agree

3. This activity was related to my nursing activity needs.
Strongly disagree   1   2   3   4   5   Strongly agree

4. The exam for the activity was an accurate test of the knowledge gained.

   Strongly disagree   1   2   3   4   5   Strongly agree

5. The activity avoided commercial bias or influence.

   Strongly disagree   1   2   3   4   5   Strongly agree

6. This activity met my expectations.

   Strongly disagree   1   2   3   4   5   Strongly agree

7. Will this learning activity enhance your professional nursing practice?

   a. Yes

   b. No

8. This educational method was an appropriate delivery tool for the nursing/clinical audience.

   Strongly disagree   1   2   3   4   5   Strongly agree

9. How committed are you to making the behavioral changes suggested in this activity?

   a. Very committed

   b. Somewhat committed

   c. Not committed

10. Please provide us with your degree

   a. ADN

   b. BSN

   c. MSN

   d. Other, please state _____

11. Please provide us with your credentials
    a. LVN
    b. LPN
    c. RN
    d. NP
    e. Other, please state _____

12. The fact that this product provides nursing contact hours influenced my decision to buy it.
    Strongly disagree   1   2   3   4   5   Strongly agree

13. I found the process of obtaining my continuing education credits for this activity easy to complete.
    Strongly disagree   1   2   3   4   5   Strongly agree

14. If you did not find the process easy to complete, which of the following areas did you find the most difficult?
    a. Understanding the content of the activity
    b. Understanding the instructions
    c. Completing the exam
    d. Completing the evaluation
    e. Other, please state:

15. How much time did it take for you to complete this activity (including reading the book and completing the exam and the evaluation)? _____

16. If you have any comments on this activity, process, or selection of topics for nursing CE, please note them below.

17. Would you be interested in participating as a pilot tester for the development of future HCPro nursing education activities?

    a. Yes

    b. No

Thank you for completing this evaluation of our nursing CE activity.